The Fertile Feast

THE FERTILE FEAST

Dr. Kiltz's Essential Guide to Keto for Fertility

DR. ROBERT KILTZ, M.D.

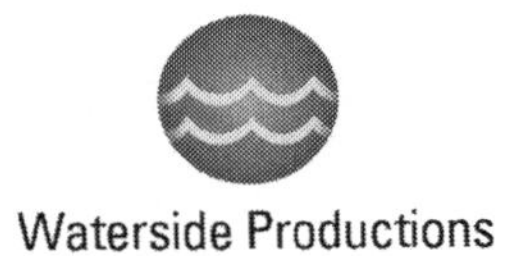

Waterside Productions

Printed in the United States of America

First Printing, 2020

ISBN-13: 978-1-949003-26-0 print edition
ISBN-13: 978-1-949003-27-7 ebook edition

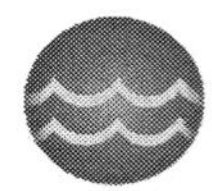

Waterside Productions

2055 Oxford Ave
Cardiff, CA 92007
www.waterside.com

Table of Contents

Introduction: The Simple Truth

During my career spanning more than two decades of helping people conceive over 20,000 babies, I've learned that for the majority of people, the most important thing in this universe is creating life. Yet all too often, I have witnessed the sad truth that Western medicine doesn't work on its own. The failure of Western medicine drove me to seek out Eastern approaches to health and wellbeing, like yoga, Tai Chi, and meditation. These tools are so effective that I've equipped my clinics with Healing Arts Centers where patients can access these practices and treatments.

But the most incredible insight I've learned over the last decade is that the foundation of our health and wellbeing, and therefore our fertility, is actually the food we eat.

Since learning the simple truth that our bodies and brains are designed to run most optimally on high-quality animal fats and that we don't need any sugar whatsoever, I have successfully recommended keto to countless patients who had previously been unable to conceive even with the combined aid of western and eastern medicines. I have witnessed the power of keto to bring new life into this world, and I have experienced it transforming my own life and the lives of my patients, friends, and colleagues.

Taking inspiration from these experiences, I created *Fertile Feast* as an essential guide to cultivating the life force I see unleashed by keto. Throughout the book, I weave keto with principles of mindful living, presenting keto as the root mantra of wellbeing and fertility.

There are a lot of keto books out there today focusing only on weight loss and improvements to physical health. I love seeing keto bring these benefits, but even more so as the gifts we receive along the journey towards our ultimate goal: *taking control of our fertility and realizing our own highest destiny in each and every moment.*

There are people who refer to keto as a diet, but to me, keto is a way of life. *Fertile Feast* is about much more than just what you put into your mouth. It's also about what you put into your mind, how you treat your body, how you feel about yourself, and how you challenge yourself to be kind, creative, and to connect with others in deep, joyous, and meaningful ways.

I became a doctor for one reason, and that's to help people. *Fertile Feast* is my guide for awakening the hidden powers of body and spirit, leading to emotional and physical healing, and a fertile life of inspiration, clarity, and joy.

-Dr. Robert Kiltz M.D.

Part I: Fertile Foundations

My Personal Path to a Keto Way of Life

"Too often we underestimate the power of a touch, a smile, a kind word, a listening ear, an honest compliment, or the smallest act of caring, all of which have the potential to turn a life around."

-Leo Buscaglia

The nutrition and lifestyle practices that I share throughout these pages are the deeply personal culmination of my three decades of medical practice and a lifetime of being me. So, I'd like to open by giving you a snapshot of the journey that has led me here to share with you my *keto way of life.*

As a teenager in East Los Angeles, I was dyslexic and could barely read. I failed classes and got kicked out of school. I was a street kid, and I'll admit it, I loved the streets. I was even in a gang—it's hard for me to say this, but it's true. And of course, I got into all kinds of trouble. At one point, my father was in jail; my sister Maryann had diabetes; my parents' businesses failed; and we lost two houses. But through it all, my parents worked hard, and despite our challenges, I always felt an unshakeable foundation of love, patience, and acceptance. These hardships combined with this love are what made it possible for me to learn from these experiences, and grow to become the doctor, and, most importantly, the person I am today.

My story, like any honestly told story, was shaped as much by the vicissitudes of fate and the people who cared about me as by anything

I myself have done or accomplished. For example, when I was sixteen, my grandmother pulled a few strings to get me my first job at a department store. Though I was failing at school, I discovered that I was an innately hard worker. I loved the long shifts that didn't let out until eleven at night. Working at the department store turned out to be one of the most important jobs in my life because it was there that I learned the power of service. In retail, it's called customer service. But from early on, I saw it as *people service.* Through the simple daily job of serving people, I realized how everyone thrives on patience, kindness, and love. Everyone deserves respect. And it's in this spirit of service that I offer the insights contained in this book.

THE POWER OF RESPECT

One night when I was driving home from the department store in my grandmother's Chevy Impala, I was pulled over by a motorcycle cop. He didn't give me a reason but went right ahead and searched the car. In the glovebox he found prescription medications belonging to my grandmother. Assuming that I was in illegal possession of prescription drugs, the officer threw me up against a chain-link fence and handcuffed me. I was pretty terrified and confused. Eventually he confirmed that the medications belonged to my grandmother and he let me go without even writing me a ticket.

When I got home, I told my father what had happened. To my surprise, my father called the police station, got in touch with the motorcycle officer directly, and asked the officer if he would come over and apologize to me. Amazingly, he agreed! I have a lot of respect for that officer and for his willingness to admit he made a mistake and show me respect. From this experience, I learned how a little vulnerability and respect can be deeply healing both for the person receiving it and the person offering it. I also learned the power of having a caring advocate in your corner—someone who knows how to stand up to injustice, but also how to speak to power in a way that creates mutual respect and healing, not just antagonism and anger. These lessons in advocacy, care, and respect are part of my DNA, and they are the motivating forces behind my exploration into the practices and insights I discuss in this book, many of which run in direct opposition to the dogmas of the mainstream medical establishment.

AS FATE WOULD HAVE IT

Though I failed algebra and English, I found a passion for pottery and art when by chance the Spanish course I wanted to get into was full. While looking for another class to fill out my schedule, I wandered into the ceramic's studio. I hadn't taken an art class since first grade, but I was immediately hooked. My ceramics teacher, Mrs. Wong, helped me discover that I was good with my hands, and I loved the deep meditative presence of controlling my body in precise ways while throwing pots on the wheel. These skills would serve me well when later I became a doctor of obstetrics and gynecology with the truly blessed job of working closely with the human body and delivering life into this world.

But back then I had no idea I would become a doctor. It wasn't even a blip on my radar until I broke my leg during my freshman year in college. This was the mid-1970s, and the family doctor who treated me was a quintessential hippy. He was friendly, warm, down to earth, and he genuinely loved helping people. Meeting this doctor was the moment when something clicked deep within me; I thought hey, this looks like a really great way to live. As a doctor, I could be an advocate in service to others, treating everyone with respect and kindness, and using emotional presence and tactile skills to truly help others.

DR. GURU

Fast forward through medical school to an early career in obstetrics, delivering babies, doing surgeries, providing primary care, to my introduction to endocrinology and in-vitro fertilization, to the founding of CNY Fertility nearly twenty years ago. Throughout these whirlwind years of medical training and into the first few years of CNY Fertility, I was a Standard American Doctor—and though I made great friends, learned a ton, benefited from generous mentors, and found fertility to be an exciting and rewarding field, the acronym "SAD" began to define my experience. All too often, the mainstream medications and procedures were failing. I had an intuitive, but not yet defined sense that the standard Western approach to treatment was missing something essential.

Then, around fifteen years ago, patients who I had previously been unable to treat successfully began getting pregnant. I asked them if anything had changed in their lives, and I discovered that these patients had begun practicing Eastern healing arts and philosophies like acupuncture, massage, yoga, and meditation. I was skeptical at first. Most of these treatments hadn't been subjected to rigorous scientific experimentation, and they weren't supported by the leading medical journals. But my first-hand observations were undeniable. So, I stepped back, watched, and thought, Jeez, it's working!

Soon I set my ego aside and began exploring and practicing these Eastern healing arts myself. I learned the profound power of meditation and spirituality to connect us to the deepest layers of our own selves and to the hearts of the other humans we encounter every day. These practices helped me to listen, learn from, and love myself and others like never before. I began offering these practices to my patients and soon people started calling me Dr. Guru. At first, I was taken aback. I was a serious medical professional after all, and these practices, though undeniably powerful, were not yet supported by Western "science." But as the successes continued, and as I witnessed my own life transforming, I realized that these healing arts and philosophies are a science! Not just of individual cell-types, organs, and biological systems, but of the whole person, the mind, body, and that indelibly human element we call spirit or soul. I began prescribing them alongside mainstream treatments, and I noticed that they were more effective when practiced in-house in our clinics. So, I equipped my clinics with CNY Healing Arts Wellness Centers, making these treatments available to all our patients.

LOW-CARB REVELATION

"Let food be thy medicine, and medicine be thy food."

-Hippocrates

For years after I spent a lot of time talking about the mind, intentions, meditation, and deepening our connection to our bodies. That's when I began *Mind Body Smile,* my personal blog where I record and share with the world my daily intentions and discussions on how we tend to our lives through our attitudes, actions, and thoughts. But back then I didn't talk about food *at all.* In hindsight, this blind-spot seems unbelievable. Though it makes sense when considering that throughout my entire medical training there had not been a single course on nutrition and health. None of my colleagues even talked about it. It was a subject as complex, personal, and thorny as politics and religion.

Then about ten years ago I began witnessing a new trend where patients who had previously tried and failed to get pregnant with every combination of Western and Eastern medicine, suddenly began to conceive. There were patients I had entirely stopped treating who called me months later to tell me they were pregnant, then again to tell me that they had given birth to healthy babies. What all these miraculous births had in common was that these patients were practicing an eating plan known as Paleo, or the "cave man diet." So, I started doing some research and discovered that Paleo is a low-carb diet based on foods similar to what people ate during the Paleolithic era, dating from around 2.5 million to the dawn of the agricultural revolution about 10,000 years ago. Typically, Paleo includes meats, fish, fruits, vegetables, nuts and seeds—foods that in the past people would get by hunting and gathering. A Paleo diet cuts out food that became common when farming emerged, especially grains, dairy products, and legumes, and most importantly for the health of modern humans, it cuts out all our processed foods.

I took this as another golden opportunity to step-back, observe, and learn everything I could about this seemingly miraculous cure for infertility. I read voraciously while experimenting with the diet on myself. I travelled deep into the low-carb diet world, and soon found my way to the high-fat, moderate protein, low-to-no-carb Ketogenic diet. The more I read about keto and its anti-inflammatory benefits, the more I discovered about inflammation, and how it's likely the root cause of our most common and deadly diseases like heart disease, cancer, and diabetes.

This link between diet, inflammation, and disease became the most exciting and powerful insight I've come across in my entire medical career. It's the difference between approaching diseases as genetic mysteries that need to be treated with expensive medications and invasive surgeries, or as metabolic disorders that can be targeted, treated, and *cured* by straightforward diet and lifestyle choices.

This discovery struck close to home after my sister Maryann died at fifty-two from diabetes, and again when my best friend Dave died at the same age from cancer. Maryann struggled to manage her diabetes since she was four years old, and though her death was not unexpected, her suffering was difficult to bear. Dave's disease, on the other hand, came out of nowhere. He was an avid runner, naturally athletic, with infectious joie *de vivre.* And as with Dave's cancer, the infertility I encounter on a daily basis is mostly unexplained. Open tubes, normal ovulation, normal sperm, but no babies! In medicine, we call these unexplainable conditions and diseases "idiopathic," a word derived from the Greek *idios* "one's own," and *pathos* "suffering." Deeming a disease idiopathic basically means we've thrown in the towel on trying to treat or even properly understand the cause, and instead we focus on the symptoms. But since discovering the link between inflammation and disease, now when I see the word "idiopathic" I think, We're *idiots!* It turns out the root cause of most disease is inflammation!

Books like Gary Taubes' *Good Calories, Bad Calories,* and Thomas Seyfried's *Cancer as a Metabolic Disease: On the Origin, Management, and Prevention of Cancer,* were hugely influential in helping me to draw the link between diet, inflammation, and infertility—among many other diseases—and helped me understand how a keto diet can reverse and cure ailments from infertility to diabetes and cancer. Taubes, along with a growing community of medical professionals, challenges the most sacred dogma of the mainstream American nutritional establishment by showing that dietary health isn't based on the quantity of calories we consume, but rather the type and quality of our calories. This new approach dismantles the myth that low-fat eating is healthy by showing that carbohydrates from processed foods, grains, rice, flour, and starchy vegetables (and I would add all vegetables because anything that's not fat or protein is a carbohydrate) are quickly converted by our digestive system into simple sugar. When this sugar enters our blood stream, it spikes our blood sugar levels. Our bodies respond to the spike by producing insulin. Insulin converts sugar into fat that we store in our cells. What this means is that *carbs and sugar are the causes of obesity, not the fat we eat.* Obesity is not the cause of our diseases! Rather, obesity is a symptom of the real cause: hyperglycemia (i.e., high blood sugar).

Dr. Seyfried's work reveals strong evidence that cancer is a metabolic disease, and *not* a genetic disease. This idea supports Otto Warburg's theory of the origin of cancer as mitochondrial dysfunction. Mitochondria are the energy factories inside our cells. Cancer results from defects in these energy factories caused by glycation—the bonding of glucose (sugar) to our cells. Mitochondrial dysfunction triggered by glycation activates oncogenes—genes that cause tumors—and deactivates tumor suppressing genes. Not surprisingly, healthy mitochondria are the ultimate tumor suppressor.

And guess what provides the optimum fuel to the mitochondria of healthy cells? Ketones! These are the compounds our bodies burn when we stop eating carbohydrates and begin eating a diet based on animal fats. When you're fueling healthy cells with ketones, you are simultaneously starving cancer cells. Cancer cells are fueled by glucose and lack the ability to derive energy from ketones due to the mitochondrial defects that make them cancer cells in the first place.

There are numerous animal studies, reports, and my own observations, showing that metabolic therapies like carb-cutting, intermittent fasting, and above all, a fat-based ketogenic diet, quickly reduce tumor growth, extend lifespans, and cure infertility in addition to all the so-called diseases of civilization: heart disease, obesity, hypertension, type 2 diabetes, epithelial cell cancers, auto-immune disease from bowel disorders to asthma, and osteoporosis.

We call these the diseases of civilization because they were almost non-existent in hunter gatherer societies. It's no coincidence that most of the diets of these disease-free hunter gatherer societies were dominated by animal fats, and of course, completely without processed carbohydrates.

THE NEW KETO FOOD PYRAMID

Yet the keto guidelines of consuming high amounts of saturated animal fats along with very few vegetables, hardly any fruits, and zero grains, runs opposite to the low-fat, mostly vegetarian and who-legrain based diet that the mainstream medical establishment has been force-feeding us since the 1960's. The new keto food pyramid completely upends the old paradigm.

Ketogenic Diet Pyramid

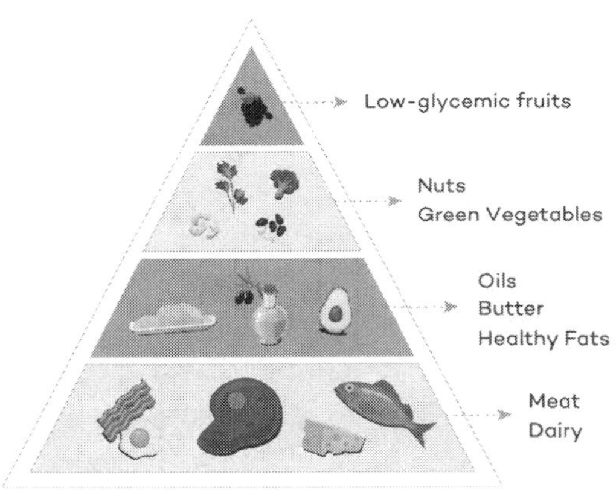

When we follow the mainstream guidelines to eat a mostly vegetarian diet for three meals a day, we're filling up our digestive tract with complex carbs, fruits and veggies chalk full of natural plant pesticides, bacteria, and microorganisms. I like to call our ubiquitous triple-washed lettuce "nature's toilet paper." Just think of all the lettuce recalls you've heard of over the years. Now try and think of a single recall for rib-eye steak. All this dirty, sugary, abrasive ruffage we're eating clogs up our digestive system, spawning yeast and bacteria that ferments into highly inflammatory alcohol and aldehyde.

The foods and fiber we're "supposed" to be eating in abundance create a constant slurry of inflammatory waste. When I examined the studies exploring the benefits of fiber and vegetables, I wasn't surprised to find that there is zero evidence demonstrating the benefits of fiber for bowel health—a revelation that I go into more detail on in later chapters. What we do know for certain is just how little we *actually* know about our complex and delicate digestive system. And this is yet another reason why I find the mainstream diet recommendations so troubling—a topic we'll dig into further.

My observations as a fertility doctor lead me to believe that the constant sugar and fiber fermenting in our bowels spreads inflammation to tissue and organs throughout the entire lower abdominal region, including our tubes, ovaries, uterus, prostate, seminal vesicles, and testicles. It bears emphasizing that in the majority of cases I treat, infertility is an inflammatory disease! And inflammation doesn't stop in the lower abdomen. Destructive plant antigens—naturally occurring vegetable compounds that attack healthy human cells—and glucose are micronized in our gut and deposited through the blood stream to every organ in our bodies. The most difficult thing about detecting inflammation is that for the most part, it's invisible. I've seen countless patients who appear physically healthy who can't conceive, and I've also seen many patients who were overweight or otherwise visibly unhealthy who conceived with little assistance.

VARIETY IS DEADLY

For decades I myself ate "healthy" salads, whole grains, and lean meats. Yet I suffered from bowel issues, kidney stones, joint and back problems. Now at sixty-three years old, I'm in the best shape of my life, and I have keto to thank for it. My most common dinner is a fatty rib-eye steak with butter. Occasionally, I'll have a few French fries fried in duck tallow or lard.

Thinking of this simple yet nutrient packed and wonderfully healthy meal brings me to another key component of my keto way of life, the part that is probably the most difficult for most people to put into practice... at first. Yet, as you'll realize when you begin, it's so obvious: The less variety we eat the better off we are. Variety is deadly. Sides are deadly. Spices are deadly.

Variety adds up to inflammation, and eating lots of different foods runs in direct opposition to the way we were evolved to eat. Remember, 100,000 years ago humans only had access to the few foods that were available in their immediate surroundings during specific seasons. We are made to fast and feast. Which is why I recommend eating only one meal a day at dinner to give your body plenty of time to rest and digest. Our bodies are meant to go days without food, hours without water, and only minutes without air. And our bodies don't need any carbohydrates whatsoever.

Our liver makes all the carbs we need from protein. The key to the benefits of keto comes from radically simplifying what we eat. As it turns out, boring is better. Keto liberates us from our addiction to the kinds of foods that keep us hunting for our next sugar fix, freeing up mental and emotional space, energy, and time for healthier pursuits like art, family, and nature. Keto helps us to become more present with all the gifts available to each and every one of us. And you don't have to take my word for it. The benefits of eating keto such as mental clarity, mood and energy stabilization, improved sleep, and general wellbeing, come on fast. The proof is in *not* eating the pudding. I've witnessed the power of keto to put diabetes into full remission in a matter of months. My own colleagues who were resistant at first have kicked chronic hyper-tension. But I've seen countless families fall prey to the invasive and expensive litany of pills, pokes, and procedures.

I like to sum up my keto way of life in a few salient lines: *We came out of the trees not to eat the grass but to eat the grass eaters!* We are fat-making and fat-eating machines. Super markets are super packed with super foods that are super damaging to us! Let's scrap the word "diet", and call keto what it is, a *live-it* plan! Keto is the most natural and effective way to heal and thrive that I've ever come across, and I'm deeply grateful to have this opportunity to share my keto way of life with you!

Karen's Story

The race to preserve my fertility has spanned ten years, and this is my story. When I was 19 years old, I had appendicitis. My CT scan prior to surgery also showed a large cyst on my right ovary the size of a tennis ball. My appendix hadn't ruptured, but instead had sprung a leak allowing a large amount of bacterial fluid into my abdomen. It was not safe to remove the large cyst at the same time, so I went in for another surgery three months later. Upon the removal of the large cyst, it was discovered that it was actually a large cluster of multiple cysts. With this surgery, I lost about half of my right ovary. I was diagnosed with polycystic ovarian syndrome. The symptoms had been there for years, but I never put two and two together. I was prescribed a different birth control pill to help manage my PCOS.

Three months later I was still having pain and discomfort and underwent yet another surgery. What had not been present only three months prior had reared its ugly head. I had an aggressive case of endometriosis to accompany my PCOS. I was also diagnosed with interstitial cystitis, so there were now multiple causes contributing to my pain. With each surgery and the fluid from appendicitis, there was more and more scar tissue invading my abdomen causing more problems from "gluing" my organs together, even further contributing to my presumed infertility.

Over the next several years, I underwent numerous treatments, switching to treat the different diseases and trying to find a balance. I did three rounds of Lupron, lasting six months each, to treat the endometriosis by putting my body in a chemically induced menopause. The last round was cut a bit short because of the side effects of the medicine on my then newly diagnosed heart condition PSVT. I had four more surgeries during this same time to remove cysts, scar tissue, and lesions from the endometriosis. This span of time was a blur of surgery, medications, and induced menopause, all of which seemed to be taking a toll on my overall health.

By age of 25, I had given up. I couldn't take anymore. Trying to preserve my fertility in any sense seemed like a hopeless cause at this point. I had just had a knee surgery for a rare tumor on top of everything else, and I just didn't have any fight left in me. I was always in pain of some sort, and as time progressed, my chances for having children continued to dwindle. I made yet another appointment for an exam, and my fears were confirmed. It was suggested that it was time to have a hysterectomy as I had run out of treatment options. I had ruptured three cysts that month and continued to have hemorrhaging on and off. I requested a two-week time period to digest the news and let them know I would call after that time to schedule the surgery.

A few days after that appointment I had a strange feeling. I looked at my high dose birth control pill pack and noticed that I was a few days late getting my period. Though this is common with these medical conditions, it was a bit less common while on the high dose of medication I was on. I took a pregnancy test, and it was positive.

I was already pregnant at the appointment, but it had been too early to show up on their urine test. With all of my surgeries coupled with my conditions, I was fearful that the pregnancy wouldn't last. I had a high-risk pregnancy, and much to my surprise, it did in fact last. At the end of the pregnancy, I got pre-eclampsia, so I was induced a week early.

After 24 hours of labor, my stats and my baby's stats started to drop, so we needed an emergency c-section. We welcomed a healthy baby boy, Ralph, in November of 2015. He was my miracle baby, something I never thought possible with all I had been through. He was a surprise pregnancy—a surprise we will forever be grateful for.

Having Ralph gave me a sense of hope about my conditions and that they might allow us to have another child. A few months after Ralph was born, I was having a different abdominal pain. I had chronical cholecystitis and needed to have my gallbladder out, yet another surgery on top of all the others including my recent c-section. My now husband and I were in the process of wedding planning when I started to have bleeding problems and pain yet again. Both the endometriosis and the PCOS were back.

Ralph was only a year old when I was informed that my time was limited to have another baby with the progression of my diseases. It wasn't ideal to think about possibly being pregnant for our upcoming wedding, but we weren't going to let that chance slip away. We tried for more than a year with no success. I did basal temperature tracking, ovulation tracking tests, counting the calendar days. Everything we could do was already being done, and nothing was working.

Having Ralph had given me a false sense of hope, and it also made me greedy. He was such an amazing addition to our lives that we wanted more of that love, and we wanted another child to complete our family.

I became discouraged, depressed, and stressed from putting so much effort and hope into getting pregnant again. I looked at various fertility clinic websites, and the prices were way out of our budget.

Then I saw CNY Fertility's website. It seemed like a good match for us feeling wise, and financially. I scheduled my appointment in January for a consultation in March. In the meantime, I joined a few of the CNY Fertility support groups suggested by one of my friends who had just successfully become pregnant with the help of CNY Fertility. It was suggested by many in the groups and from Dr. K's video chats that I start the strict Keto diet while waiting for my consultation.

The strict Keto diet of beef, butter, bacon, and eggs was a challenge to adapt to. To start, I gave myself a little bit of leeway with some additional foods consisting of avocado, cheese, heavy cream, naturally cured Italian meats, and a little bit of Bibb lettuce dipped in oil and vinegar when I needed a palate cleanser so to speak to break up the heaviness of the BEBBI diet. Two weeks into the diet I felt successful in achieving the transition. I felt great! My skin was clearer, my psoriasis better, asthma improved, I had more energy, I wasn't in pain, I hadn't ruptured an ovarian cyst recently, and I was losing weight even though I hadn't cut my calories. I was detailing my diet successes with another person in one of the Facebook groups when something clicked. There were too many good changes for them all to be from the diet.

I had one pregnancy test left. It was too early to be testing that month, and I was more focused on getting started on the diet so we hadn't put much effort into conceiving that month. I took the test anyway; I was discouraged before I even looked at it because of all the previous negatives I had seen. I went to just throw the test out, but then I thought I'd be wasting money if I didn't at least look at it. So, I looked at it, and it was positive. I was shocked, my heart was racing, and I was in complete disbelief.

My first month of starting the BEBBI diet was successful. This diet did what more than a year of everything else could not: it allowed us to conceive without much effort.

My family all thought I was crazy for pursuing this diet and lifestyle change to try to conceive, but I was willing to do anything that might give us a chance to have another baby. I had to cancel my consultation appointment before having the pleasure of meeting the CNY Fertility staff.

We had a successful pregnancy despite getting gestational diabetes this time around. In November of 2018, I had a C-section at 39 weeks during which we welcomed a beautiful baby girl named Ruby. I am complete because of CNY Fertility. The void I felt and the emotional strain from trying to conceive is gone because of Dr. K. Despite not meeting him, I followed the advice from his chats and the support groups made up of his current patients, and it worked for us. What I thought would never be possible became a reality, and I am forever thankful. I have PCOS and endometriosis, and I now have two beautiful children. It took 10 years of suffering to get to this point, but it was well worth the wait and the pain.

It is possible, and I hope that in sharing our story someone else might find that last bit of strength to continue their fertility journey and try something different because without the BEBBI diet, I wouldn't have been able to write it.

What is Keto Anyway?

"Through living a ketogenic lifestyle, the entire picture of 'me' comes into focus."

-Robert Kiltz M.D.

Around ten years ago I noticed something incredible happening at my fertility practice. I had patients who had been struggling to get pregnant for years, then on their own, they changed their diets by eliminating carbs and sugar, and suddenly they were pregnant! This diet-based fertility success seemed miraculous. But the results from my patients were enough to spark my own reading and experimenting with the Paleogenic diet—which was popular at the time. As I journeyed deeper into the low-carb diet world, I found my way to keto. I was blown away by keto's revolutionary emphasis on the undeniable benefits of fat. I didn't believe it at first; *Fat is good for you?* This shook the foundations of everything I had been taught in my medical training and as a practitioner of healthy living. But there were those patients calling me months after I had stopped treating them to tell me they were pregnant. So, I tried keto for myself and I've never looked back. Since then I've made it my life's work to share this incredible insight: The foundation of our health and wellbeing, and therefore our fertility, is the food we eat!

In the decade since I first discovered the power of keto to promote fertility, I have recommended the diet to thousands of people, including patients, friends, and family. Yet, at first, I'm almost always met with disbelief. How in the world can saturated fat be healthy? What do you mean I should cut out fruit and fiber? I get it. I had the same reaction. It was imperative for me that I understand as much as I could about keto before I felt comfortable recommending it to everyone I know. I'd like to share with you what I discovered. Now let's take it from the top (of the food chain).

LET'S TAKE IT FROM THE TOP (OF THE FOODCHAIN)

We humans are apex predators. As we evolved from earlier primates, we came down from the security of the forest canopy, left behind a vegetarian diet of leaves and fruits, and began hunting and eating meat. Then, for the vast majority of human history—we're talking hundreds of thousands of years—we lived as hunter gatherers. As hunter gatherers, our diets consisted mostly of wild meats, and to a lesser degree on gathered nuts and fruits. By 'meats' I mean the whole animal, and especially the fat and organs. We see historical evidence for the prizing of fat over lean muscle meat in numerous anthropological accounts of tribes savoring the fattiest morsels and throwing tenderloins and other lean parts to the dogs, or simply leaving them to scavengers. Not surprisingly, we see the same behavior by lions—the other apex predators—on the African savannah. When we're talking about eating "meat," we're primarily talking about eating fat. Meat is made up exclusively of fat, protein, and minerals, and contains zero carbohydrates i.e. sugars.

This is significant because our pre-human ancestors lived almost exclusively on carbohydrates. So, in order for humans to get energy from a fatty, meat-based diet, we had to evolve an ability to break down fatty-acids into molecules called ketone bodies that supply energy to our most crucial organs including our brain, heart, and muscles.

THE ABC's OF KETOSIS

We call this process of getting energy from fat, ketosis. If you're of a technical mind, I'll explain how this works over the next few sentences. If you don't care about the chemistry of it, feel free to jump ahead.

To turn fat into fuel our bodies take acetyl CoA, a molecule that is normally oxidized into water and CO_2 as part of the citric acid cycle, and convert it in the liver into acetoacetate and 3-hydroxybutyrate (BHB), the two most common ketone bodies. These ketones are now free to flow through the blood and lymphatic systems to everywhere they're needed in the body. Compared with glucose—the molecule that fuels our bodies when we're not burning fat—ketones are like high-octane racing fuel for our cells. By comparison, 100 grams of glucose generates 8.7 kg of ATP (ATP is the energy used most readily by our cells). Whereas 100 g of 3-hydroxybutyrate yields 10.5 kg of ATP, and 100 g of acetoacetate 9.4 kg of ATP. It's no surprise then that most parts of our bodies, including our brains, prioritize ketones over glucose whenever possible. For the remaining processes that still need glucose for energy, the liver converts non-carbohydrate sources such as fatty acids from protein into the perfect amount of glucose.

Ketosis Explained!

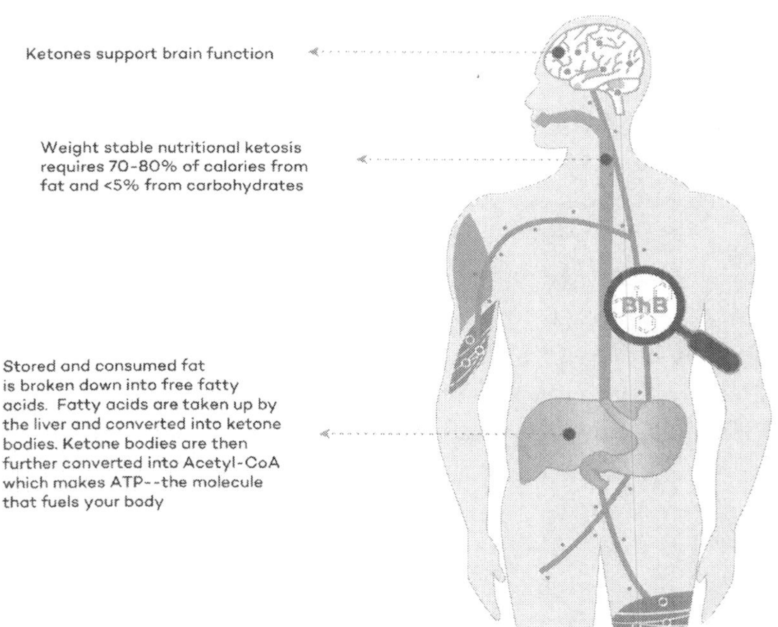

Ketones support brain function
Weight stable nutritional ketosis requires 70-80% of calories from fat and <5% from carbohydrates
BhB
Stored and consumed fat is broken down into free fatty acids. Fatty acids are taken up by the liver and converted into ketone bodies. Ketone bodies are then further converted into Acetyl-CoA which makes ATP--the molecule that fuels your body

Evolving this process of ketosis was equally crucial for the development and survival of our species when we began eating mostly meat, as when we were forced to fast during periods between successful hunts. These periods lasted anywhere from days to weeks. When we're in a fasting state, our bodies use our own fat stores for fuel, which is why most of us have a tendency to carry around a spare tire or a plump backside. These physical features are the human version of the humps on a camel's back, which, *surprise,* aren't filled with water, but with fat! Many scientists believe that the majority of hunter gatherer societies spent significant and extended periods of time in ketosis. What this means is that ketosis is the metabolic state that our bodies are most optimally and naturally designed for.

RUNNING ON CARBS IS RUNNING ON EMPTY

When you're getting more than 10% of your calories from carbohydrates your body does not go into ketosis. Instead it runs on glucose. All the cells in your body get their fuel by taking sugar from your bloodstream. Yet you only have about a teaspoon of sugar in your bloodstream at one time, so you have to refuel by devouring more and more carbs. It's as though you're constantly running on empty, always on the lookout for a gas station, and you never have more than a couple of bucks in your pocket. All this consumption of sugar is filling your bowels with fibrous junk that ferments into aldehyde and alcohol damaging your intestines and causing inflammation throughout your entire body. While at the same time you're consuming more sugar than is safe for your blood to handle.

Because high blood sugar damages your cells, your body is working hard to remove the excess sugar as quickly as possible. To keep your sugar levels in check, your liver produces a constant stream of insulin that turns the sugar into fat that's stored on your body. But just as soon as the initial flood of excess sugar is turned into fat, your body begins to run out of the limited sugar in the blood stream, so your cells scream out to be doused with ever more sugar.

You get tired, hungry, irritable, distracted. Then you have to manually adjust your blood sugar by eating. The cycle goes on and on.

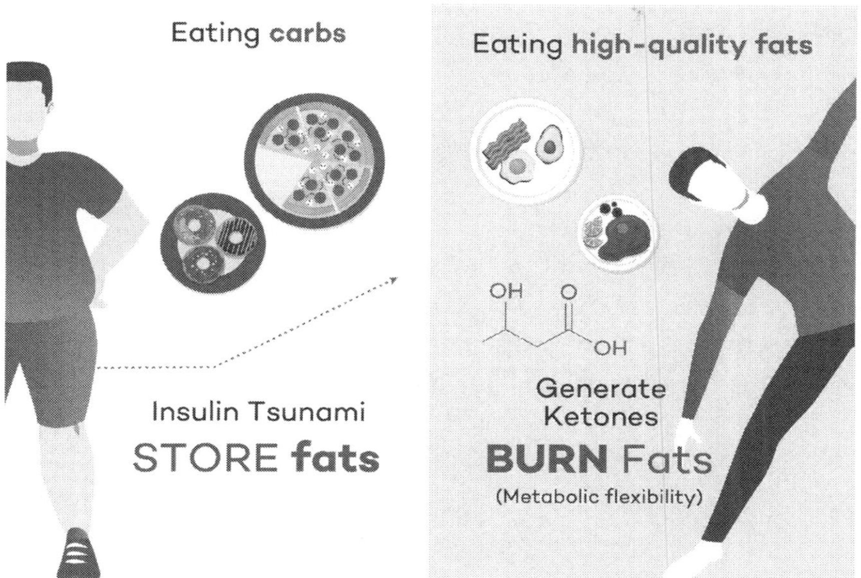

KETO PUTS YOUR METABOLISM ON AUTO-PILOT

When you're running on ketones your body naturally and efficiently regulates your blood sugar with precision. Most of the cells in your body run optimally on ketones which they get from the fat you eat as well as the fat already stored in your body. The few cell types that do require sugar are fed by glucose that your liver creates on-demand out of protein. This is why when you're on keto you can be completely satiated by eating only one meal a day. Your body demands much less sugar from your blood, resulting in remarkably steady energy and clear mental functioning. Keto is like flipping on the auto-pilot switch to your metabolism. Your liver turns fat into ketones, and protein into glucose with optimal efficiency.

By contrast, when you're on a sugar-based diet, the capacity of your liver to store the right amount of sugar is overwhelmed. Your liver has to turn the excess sugar into fat, and your body rarely turns this stored fat into ketones. So, when considering the efficiency of keto, and the inefficiency of carbohydrates, I believe that we are evolved to be in a state of keto as often as possible. The best way we can treat our DNA—the building blocks of every cell in our bodies—is by feeding it the foods that over millennia it has come to expect, and therefore use most efficiently. We are perfectly tuned machines engineered and honed by nature and time. Keto is our perfect fuel.

Yet nowadays, with grocery stores and fast food available on every corner, it's difficult to fight the primal urge to refuel, often to excess, and almost always on carbohydrates—everything that's not fat or protein is a carbohydrate, including grains, veggies, legumes, and fruits. In order to kick our bodies into ketosis we have to simulate the macro nutrient intake of our ancestors by dramatically changing our diets.

Ketogenic Diet Breakdown

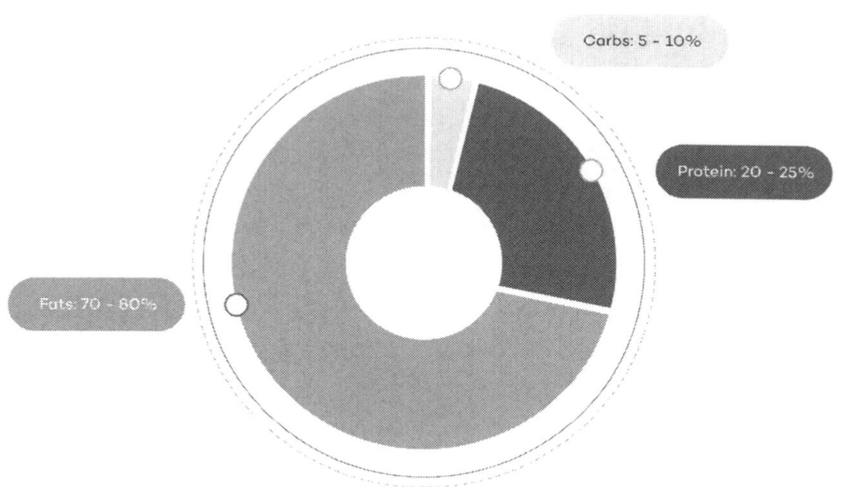

A typical American diet is about 65% carbohydrates, 15% protein, and 20% fat. Whereas the typical keto diet means we're eating around 70-75% fat, 20-25% protein, and 5-10% carbohydrates. With my *Kiltz's Keto Cure,* I take it a step further by suggesting a macro nutrient intake of 80% fat, 20% protein, and 0% carbohydrates.

THE HUMAN FERRARI

A metaphor that I find helpful to bring this all home is to think of your body as a human Ferrari. We seldom take the time to marvel at the incredible design and engineering of the human body. It is truly a wondrous thing. I call it the human Ferrari because like the revered Italian-designed sports car, our bodies are beautiful machines impeccably designed to do marvelous things. Each one of us is exquisite in both our design and function.

It has been my experience, as both a physician and diligent observer of human nature, that we humans show more appreciation and concern for the high-priced sports car than we do for our own bodies. We treat the Ferrari with kid gloves, polishing them, giving them the best gas and oil, and driving them cautiously. Yet we treat our Human Ferraris with complete disregard. We put the wrong fuel in our tank—sugar, carbs, alcohol and harmful ideas in our minds, creating cycles of shame, unworthiness, and consequently a desire for temporary satisfactions that fail to make us happy. Then we try to feel better by literally wearing out our bodies with high-impact exercises and constant stress. We're treating our beautiful, expensive, irreplaceable, and amazing bodies like rental cars, or worse, Yugos, that much maligned other Italian-designed automobile that was the butt of many jokes and regarded as the lemon of the auto industry. Yet we have the ability to change all of this! With my keto way of life, we can treat our bodies like the invaluable creations they are.

We are all human Ferraris. We all have the same blueprint and high-quality parts. There's nothing stopping us from being a sleek, powerful machine but our intentions and our habits. I hear people blame genetics for everything under the sun: why you can't lose weight, why it's likely you'll become diabetic, get arthritis, etc. I must respectfully disagree.

We all have essentially the same genetics. If you put every cell of your body under a microscope and compared it to mine, they would look no different. Yes, your DNA codes for different things like eye color, hair color, skin color, and height, but our genetics are 99.9% the same. What I've found while developing my keto way of life is that what we are putting into our bodies and our minds makes the difference between health and wellness, disorder and disease.

You have the power to change your diet in a way that will change your life. I've seen countless people take control of their destinies by cutting carbs and basing their diets on healthy fats. I've watched people kick insulin, hypertension, and cholesterol meds. Chronic bowel diseases like IB and Ulcerated Colitis have gone into full remission. Skin disorders like eczema clear up. And for the first time in peoples' lives, they feel at home in their own bodies. I invite you to discover these benefits for yourselves by journeying with me into a keto way of life.

KETO THROUGH THE AGES

Keto has been around as long as humans have walked the earth. This is because keto is not really a diet, it's a (metabolic) state of being. We've touched on keto's prevalence among hunter gatherer societies i.e. *all human societies* for the vast majority of time. But the first record of ketosis as a therapy was by Hippocrates, Greek doctor, and "father of medicine," around 400 B.C.

Before Hippocrates came along, the Greeks believed that epilepsy was a kind of spiritual possession doled out as punishment by the moon goddesses Selene and Artemis. This belief is preserved in the word epilepsy itself, derived from the Greek *epilēpsia,* meaning to seize or take hold of. Because epilepsy was of divine origin, it was believed to be so powerful it could not be healed.

Then Hippocrates came along with his radical approach to medicine where he based his practice on observations and on the study of the human body. Regarding epilepsy, he took the position that, "It is not, in my opinion, any more divine or more sacred than other diseases, but has a natural cause, and it's supposed divine origin is due to men's inexperience." In his book *Of the Epidemics*, Hippocrates applies this approach to the case of a man who was racked by seizures for five days. After prescribing that the man fast, on day six Hippocrates observed that "abstained from everything, both gruel and drink, there were no further seizures." Though he didn't have the tools or knowledge of neuroscience to completely understand why fasting worked, Hippocrates revealed the power of fasting to produce ketones that prevent epilepsy.

His discovery is echoed 500 years later, of all places, in the bible. Mark 9:14-29 of the King James bible tells the story of Jesus walking through town when he notices a crowd arguing. Seeing his disciples in the crowd, Jesus walks over.

"What are you arguing with them about?" he asks.

A man answers, "Teacher, I brought you my son, who is possessed by a spirit that has robbed him of speech. Whenever it seizes him, it throws him to the ground. He foams at the mouth, gnashes his teeth and becomes rigid. I asked your disciples to drive out the spirit, but they could not." As accurate an account of seizure as one can write.

"Bring the boy to me," says Jesus.

The boy is stricken by another crippling seizure.

Jesus turns to the boy and commands, "Come out of him and never enter him again."

The spirit shrieks and leaves the boy. Jesus takes the boy by the hand and lifts him to his feet.

Later Jesus's disciples ask, "Jesus, why couldn't we drive it out?"

Jesus replies, "This kind can come out only by prayer and *fasting*."

THE (RE)DISCOVERY OF KETO

These ancient guys didn't have the scientific knowledge of the body and neuroscience that we have today, but because keto is so fundamental to our physiology, they didn't need it.

Remarkably, we still don't fully understand the complex mechanisms by which keto cures epilepsy. But that's the beauty of keto. It is so much a part of how we are designed that all we have to do is flip the metabolic switch from burning sugar to burning fat—in these early cases by fasting—and the results speak for themselves. But despite these early accounts, fasting as a therapy seems to have gone underground during the dark ages, and didn't emerge again until the 20th century.

In the Victorian era, the standard medical belief was that epilepsy was caused by masturbation, and the way to prevent seizures was to kill off people's libidos by prescribing the powerful sedative potassium bromide. Though this treatment did a passable job of controlling seizures, it nearly killed the patients themselves, rendering them sick and lifeless. And it goes without saying that there is no link between masturbation and epilepsy! Yet this treatment persisted until 1911 when French Physicians Guelpa and Marie, conducted the first scientific report on the power of fasting to effectively treat epilepsy.

Across the pond in the 1920's, researchers at Johns Hopkins University and the Mayo Clinic searching for ways to treat intractable seizures and diabetes, discovered that fasting alleviated and even cured their patients' symptoms. But since fasting was not a long-term option— if you don't eat for long enough you die! —they tinkered with ways to simulate the fasting state by reducing carbs to almost zero. This produced higher levels of ketones in their patients—the state called ketosis. Dr. Wilder of the Mayo clinic identified ketosis as the root of the diet's restorative power, and the ketogenic diet was born.

Yet with the advent of newer more effective epilepsy drugs that could control seizures without requiring disciplined diets, keto remained a fringe treatment for decades. Then in 1994, the ketogenic diet was featured on NBC's Dateline show, marking its mainstream debut. The Dateline story follows Charlie Abrahams, a two-year-old ravaged by epilepsy despite all the drugs and therapies his five pediatric neurologists, two homeopathic physicians, a faith healer, and his parents could provide. That was until Jim, Charlie's father, happened upon a decades old reference to the early Johns Hopkins studies. At his wit's end, the father started his son on the keto diet and the seizures disappeared! Alarmed and rightfully pissed off that nobody had told them about the healing power of a simple change in diet, Jim took it upon himself to spread the good word on keto. He created the Charlie Foundation to share info with doctors and parents. He also happened to be a Hollywood director, so he took it upon himself to make the 1997 film *First Do No Harm* starring Meryl Streep, telling the story of an epileptic boy cured by keto. This popular exposure triggered a spike in keto interest, at least among medical professionals. After Charlie's Dateline episode, the number of published research papers on Keto surged from an average of just 4 per year to 40 per year.

But it wasn't until November 3, 2015, when a fateful podcast of the *Tim Ferris Show* with keto researcher Dr. Dom D'Agostino rocketed keto from relative obscurity to the top of Google news. And the momentum is still building. In 2018, keto became the number one diet trend on Google, 300% more popular than the second-place Mediterranean diet. Searches for Keto hit 17 million per month, and Orian Research estimates keto to be a $5 billion industry and growing.

Yet, despite keto's buzz and a slew of new research supporting its benefits, for the average American, the keto way of life can be really difficult to wrap your head around. Consuming high amounts of saturated animal fats along with very few vegetables, hardly any fruits, and zero grains, runs opposite to the low-fat, mostly vegetarian and wholegrain based diet that the mainstream medical establishment has been force-feeding us since the 1960's. That's why when I'm asked the question *what is keto anyway?* one of my short answers is, "Keto is a complete contradiction to the traditional food pyramid."0

THE RAISIN BRAN PARADOX

Believe me, I understand how difficult it is to turn your back on the recommendations of the powerful healthcare-agricultural-industrial-complex. Since we were kids, we've been bombarded with bad information and false branding. Ever notice those "Heart Healthy" badges on boxes of cereal? They're bought and sold by lobbyists working for giant food companies in cahoots with influential careerist medical professionals and ill-informed politicians.

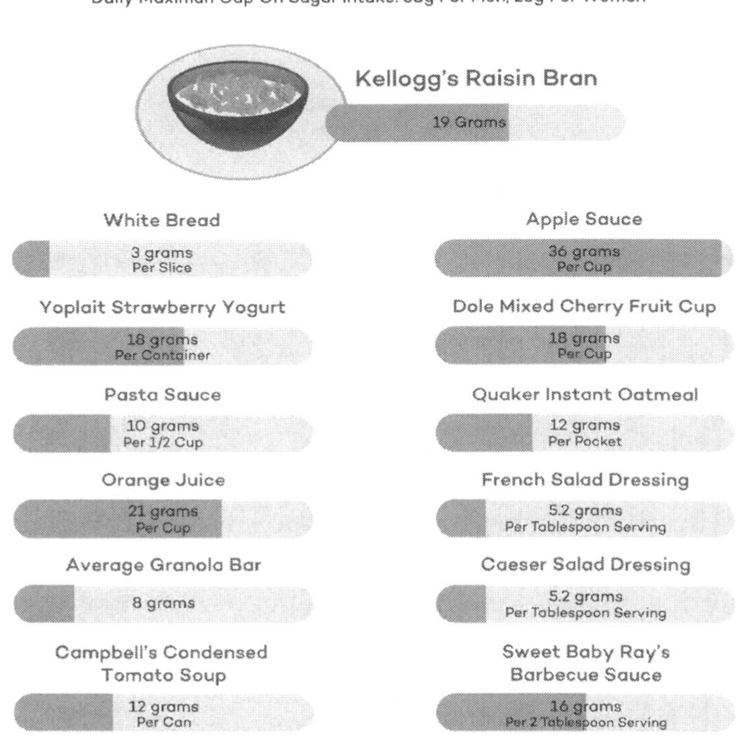

Take for example Kellogg's Raisin Bran. For decades it was the gold standard of healthy breakfast cereal. One serving of Raisin Bran has a whopping 19 grams of sugar, just one gram shy of a Cadbury Crème Egg. Add skim milk, and you're way over. Then there's the crooked idea that one serving is just one cup of cereal. Do you know anyone who eats only one cup of cereal at a time? Me neither. Most people eat two and three times the "official" serving size. Hidden in your "heart healthy" cereal can easily be three Cadbury Crème Eggs worth of sugar! Every doctor knows sugar causes obesity and diabetes, which skyrockets your risk for heart disease. Yet Raisin Bran gets to carry a federally endorsed label advertising heart health. You don't have to be a medical professional to see there's something dangerously wrong with mainstream dietary recommendations and how their marketed to the public.

Add to this proliferation of false-advertising the endless cycle of "weight loss" plans based on low fat diets, will-power restraint, reduced portions, grueling exercise, and it's no wonder these diets fail. And when they fail, we all too often blame ourselves and fall into cycles of shame that leave us scrambling for the next fad diet based on false information, compelling us to shell out money to nutritional experts stuck in the ideology of backwards 1960's science, while we brutalize our bodies with the latest workout regimen that's more intense than the last. Just because the U.S. Marines do it doesn't mean it's good for you. Actually, it means just the opposite!

Another answer I have for people who ask me, what is keto anyway? I say, keto is an end to the madness. With all these powerful interests out there manipulating people for their own gains, getting people to believe in keto can feel more like cult deprogramming than the simple act of offering straightforward advice backed by science and medicine.

A BRIEF INTRO TO MACRONUTRIENTS

So, the first step to my keto way of life is forgetting all the conventional "wisdom" you've been taught about what you're supposed to eat. Step two is getting acquainted with the foundation of metabolic science, which I chalk-up to the fact that our bodies need exactly four things to thrive and survive: fat, water, adequate protein, and lots of oxygen. There's something glaringly absent from this list: *carbs.* You do not need any carbohydrates in your diet whatsoever. None. Zero. Zilch. In scientific terms, carbohydrates are "non-essential." This means that your body can make the glucose it needs from carbon, hydrogen, nitrogen and oxygen atoms—all of which it gets from the fat and protein we eat. However, fat and protein are *essential,* meaning your body cannot synthesize them, and you need to eat plenty of fat and protein because they are critical for your cellular functioning.

THE LYMPHATIC SYSTEM: OVERLOOKED YET ESSENTIAL

When we talk about health and wellness, people don't spend much time discussing the lymphatic system, yet it is critical to maintaining optimal health. When we eat fat, it lubricates the lymphatics, and acts like a solvent within the gut to micronize, capture and filter (via the lymph nodes) the waste residue that is brought in through the foods we eat. If we don't eat fat, many of those antigens get stuck in your gut where they can get into the submucosal layer and interstitial layer of the GI tract leading to inflammation. While other antigens are delivered to the liver where they interfere with the blood system and pollute every nook and cranny of our bodies. This is an essential part of why a high carbohydrate / low fat diet is deadly. Sugar causes glycation in the lymph system. And since the lymph system does not have smooth muscle to help propel the lymphatic fluid, it relies on the natural flow and pressure of a system that's intact and lubricated by quality fat. Lymphangitis, lymph node swelling, lymphomas, and leukemia are rampant worldwide because of a low fat / high carb diet filled with excessive frequency, volume, and variety of sugar and carbohydrates.

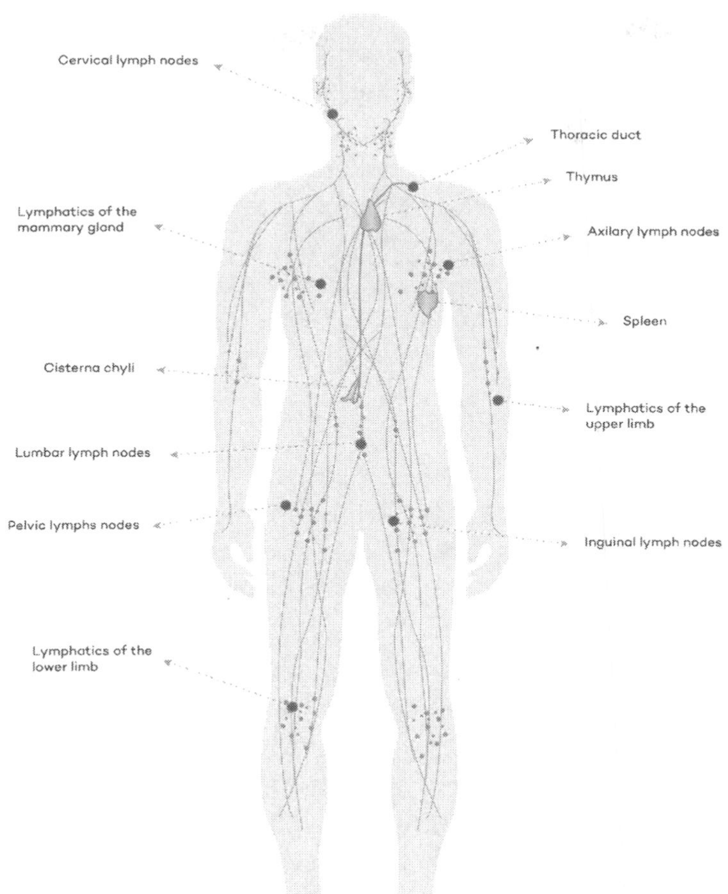

FEAR NOT CHOLESTEROL

Over the past several decades cholesterol has gotten a bad rap. Fear of high cholesterol levels on blood work panels during annual physicals erroneously steered us away from eating eggs and fatty meats, and toward lean proteins and man-made fats like margarine and vegetable oil. Yet the truth is that eggs, fatty meats, and butter don't raise cholesterol levels in our bodies. Diets high in sugar and carbs do. Our bodies need cholesterol to function correctly. Cholesterol helps us to maintain proper hormone function, and recent studies show that cholesterol is a powerful anti-oxidant. Our livers make 75% of the cholesterol we need, and it's up to us to get the other 25% from high-quality animal sources in our diets.

The true picture of how cholesterol correlates with heart disease is more complicated than simply having "high" or "low" cholesterol levels, or even with our levels of "good" HDL, or "bad" LDL. Risk for heart disease is more accurately associated with a subtype of small LDL particles floating around in your bloodstream called LDL-p. Tests for LDL-p are becoming much more common. IF you're concerned about your cholesterol levels, ask specifically for an LDL-p test.

Research shows that on keto diets HDL are likely to rise as triglycerides go down. At the same time, even though total LDL tends to stay the same, LDL-p, or particle size, tends to increase, while LDL-c or the number of particles tend to go down. This means that though the keto diet may increase your overall cholesterol level—which has essentially no bearing on heart-health—it leads to an improvement in the type of cholesterol particles that do correlate with heart health.

Looking beyond cholesterol, a much more accurate metric for understanding your risk for heart disease is your calcium, or CAC, score. Getting your calcium score can be much cheaper than getting your LDL-p—often around $100. A CAC score measures the plaque buildup in your coronary arteries, which correlates with heart disease and risk of death by many orders of magnitude more than your cholesterol score.

KETO: THE SECRET FOUNDATION OF HEALTH

On a ketogenic diet your body burns fat even while you're sleeping. It's the only diet I know of where you can literally do nothing and get skinnier and healthier. However, I want to emphasize here that when

I consider the restorative power of keto, I see weight loss as only one of keto's many benefits. In my experience as a fertility doctor and as a long-time practitioner of conscious living, I have come to believe that keto is the secret foundation for our most physically healthy, mentally clear, emotionally present, and creatively fulfilling lives. Not to mention our fertility! The very thing that keeps our species going.

One great thing about the rising popularity of keto is that it has sparked a slew of recent studies showing how keto restores the whole person, body, and mind. I believe that when our bodies and minds are balanced, we can get in touch with our souls—that beautiful space in all of us that allows us to connect to each other and the world in more open, loving, and creative ways.

So, let's take a closer look at the interconnected benefits of keto:

- **Reduced inflammation.** I believe that infertility along with the so-called diseases of civilization, are all caused by inflammation, a position I expand on later. For me, the ability of keto to dramatically reduce inflammation is its superpower. Keto works to reduce inflammation by cutting out the plant antigens and phytochemicals you ingest by eliminating vegetables, fruits, and grains from your diet. Additionally, recent studies have found that hydroxybutyrate (BHB), one of the ketones produced in abundance by your body when you are following my keto way of life, has powerful anti-inflammatory effects with positive implications for many inflammation related auto-immune diseases and disorders such as PCOS, endometriosis, arthritis, eczema, IBS, colitis, and infertility, among others. Because of the high fat basis of keto, you ingest healthier, poly-unsaturated fatty acids (PUFAs), such as DHA and EPA. These are fats you can get from quality animal sources or buy over-the-counter as brain boosting supplements. PUFAs reduce oxidation and inflammation.

- **Mental clarity and neural restoration**. The positive effects of a brain running on keto were first discovered when a carb-restricted diet was used to successfully treat children with drug resistant epilepsy. Now, with the emergence of keto into popular culture, there's been a renewed interest in studying the effects of keto on the brain. The results are inspiring to say the least. For a long time, we've known that large portions of our brains can be fueled by ketones, especially BHB. Recent studies show that BHB is a more efficient fuel than glucose, providing greater energy per unit of oxygen. This is wonderful news because what a wide range of neurological diseases from dementia to epilepsy have in common is a deficiency in energy production.

We're discovering that keto increases the "energy factory" parts of brain cells called mitochondria. This increase occurs in many areas of the brain and crucially in the hippocampus—the part of the brain responsible for learning and memory. When the hippocampus is ravaged by age-related, degenerative diseases like Alzheimer's, people suffer cognitive impairment and memory loss. The good news is that the energy produced by keto can defend against disease stressors that would otherwise wear-out and kill brain cells.

Another way keto protects and restores our mental functions is by dramatically reducing your intake of carbohydrates. When carbohydrates are broken down, they produce highly reactive and harmful oxidants. These oxidant molecules act like hordes of little Tasmanian devils banging into our proteins and membranes, damaging the fundamental structure of our physiology. The keto combination of healthy fats and drastically reduced carbohydrates greatly decreases the number of oxidants in our bodies. This reduction protects the neurons in our brains along with cells in every other part of our bodies.

The positive results from these recent studies have led to more research on the therapeutic use of keto for other neurological disorders, including migraines, brain cancer, various neurodegenerative diseases, sleep problems, bipolar disorders, and autism.

- **Reduced hunger.** Hunger is public enemy number one when it comes to other diets that rely on eating less and burning more calories. To be clear here, when I say, "other diets," I mean every other diet that isn't keto! Keto is unique in its focus on eating fat. And fat is supremely satiating. If you don't believe me, go ask the lions lolling around the African savannah after gorging on prey.

A whopping 95% of people who attempt a conventional, calorie restrictive diet, gain all their weight back—and often more—within five years. This work-your-ass-off and gain it back phenomenon isn't just because it's hard to resist eating when you're hungry, especially after grueling exercise when your body is crying out for replenishment. It's an automatic survival response to starvation that works in two ways: Your body unleashes a powerful dose of hunger hormones including ghrelin and leptin. Ghrelin causes you to crave high calorie, high-carbohydrate foods that make you as fat as possible as fast as possible. At the same time your leptin levels plummet. Leptin is the hormone that tells you when you feel full. Put these together and conventional diets are a recipe for over-eating the wrong kinds of foods, not to mention a tremendous amount of stress while trying to resist your body's most basic and persistent urges.

But even if you have the resolve of a gladiator and can will your way through starvation, cravings, and relentless hunger in order to shed a few pounds, your body will inevitably wrestle back control. Losing significant body weight on a conventional diet (10% or more) automatically triggers your metabolism to slow down. Studies show that once this calorie conserving survival mode kicks in, people begin burning 30 to 40 percent less calories per day.

Just as your body evolved in a hunter-gatherer environment to optimally produce all of its energy from metabolizing fat and protein, your body is also evolved to hold onto its fat stores in case of periods of fasting. There's no way for your body to know about the super market shelves full of high calorie junk, or the apps on your smartphone beckoning you to order any food you can imagine to your doorstep in a matter of minutes. To understand why conventional diets fail, you have to realize that *your body evolved to always be in survival mode,* optimizing its metabolic processes for a hunter-gatherer lifestyle in an environment where food was often unreliable. We're still in that same survival mode in our modern world of overabundance and easy access.

What makes keto special and sets it apart from conventional diets is that it does not require restricting your calories. Many people who begin keto find it helpful to count calories only in order to make sure they are eating *more* rather than less high-quality fats and proteins. When your body is burning healthy fats as opposed to sugars for fuel, keto subverts the body's starvation mechanism that would otherwise cause you to feel hungry and burn fewer calories.

A recent study of Australians who lost at least 13% of their body weight on keto showed they experienced zero rise in their ghrelin levels. Additionally, when on keto, most people instinctively eat fewer calories because fat is far more satiating than carbohydrates, takes longer to digest, and releases energy more slowly, causing you to feel fuller faster, and giving you more energy while keeping you less hungry for longer. Say goodbye to the carbohydrate rollercoaster of energy peaks and dips, and feel the liberation when you're no longer searching like a zombie for your next carbohydrate fix.

HONOR THYSELF

By following my *keto way of life,* you are honoring the ways your body was optimized to eat over tens of thousands of generations. Our hunter-gatherer ancestors were adapted to a mode of survival that was designed for a different environment than we live in today. Yet we share the same genetics. This means that you and I are always in survival mode, and that we are evolved to thrive on a narrow spectrum of macronutrients. My plan of wholesome, high-quality foods providing 70-80% of your calories from fat, 20% from protein, and hardly any from carbs is a way to align with the past as it is alive within us, as us! While at the same time protecting our minds and bodies from the modern, mortal-threats of effortless access to industrially processed and high-carbohydrate foods. My keto plan will help you look your best, achieve robust and lasting health, increase your fertility and give you the energy and inspiration to live your very best life.

YOU ARE THE KINGS AND QUEENS OF THE JUNGLE. EAT LIKE IT!

When I'm introducing my keto way of life to patients and friends, I often say that going keto is to eat like a lion or lioness—the kings and queens of the jungle. We humans are not lowly herbivores meant to graze all day on grass, grain, fruits, vegetables, and fibers. *We came out of the trees to eat the grass eaters, not to eat the grass!*

Rachel's Story

Dr. Kiltz,

My name is Rachel. My husband and I had a consult over the phone with you in August. You may not remember us, but we will always remember that conversation. It changed our lives. The day after the consult I began following your recommended Keto diet, resting my body and reading the word of the Lord. A short time after, in October, we found out we were pregnant! I am now 5 months pregnant and due in June! Although we have never met face-to-face, we cannot thank you enough for your knowledge and time. It is clear that you are very knowledgeable and passionate about helping people. We had a long an emotional fertility journey. I only wish we would have met you sooner. Once again, thank you!

Forever grateful,
Rachel

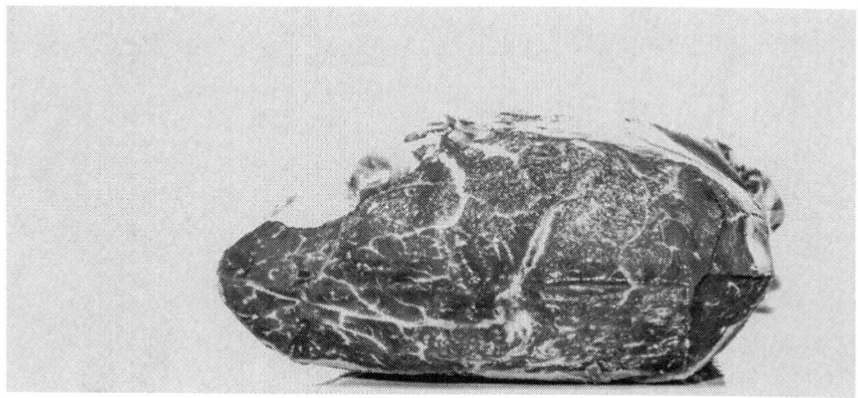

For humans to eat like lions means a diet based on bacon, eggs, butter, and beef, and occasionally full fat ice-cream. Later in this book I offer a vegetarian keto option because I believe keto is for everyone. But for me, the healthiest and most effective keto meal plans are based on animal fats. I consider a rib-eye steak to be the perfect keto food, and it's one I eat quite often. Rib-eyes have a high fat content, and generally, the higher the grade of meat, the more fat it contains. A high-quality rib-eye has a ratio of half fat and half protein in one delicious package, and it contains no carbohydrates, sugar, or fiber. To meet my macronutrient fat to protein ratio, I'll add butter and tallow to the rib-eye, making it even more delicious and satiating. About 40 percent of the fat in a rib-eye comes from saturated fat, including essential fatty acids that the body can't produce on its own. These fatty acids reduce inflammation, control blood clotting, and aid in brain function. Fat also allows the body to absorb vitamins A, D, E and K. A serving of rib-eye steak offers 239% of the recommended daily intake of vitamin B12 for an adult male. Vitamin B12 helps red blood cell formation, neurological health, DNA synthesis, and may play a role in reducing the risks of dementia and age-related cognitive decline. Rib-eye steak also provides 84% of your daily recommended intake of niacin, which helps in red blood cell formation, neurological function, and maintaining healthy digestion, skin health and nerve function. This same serving of rib-eye supplies 153% of your daily need for zinc. Zinc is integral to energy production, protein and nucleic acid synthesis, healthy immune function, and cell division. You also get 145% of the daily requirement for selenium. Selenium combines with proteins to form antioxidant selenoproteins that help prevent cellular damage from free radicals, which studies suggest can lower cancer and heart disease risks. Selenium may also play a role in alleviating arthritis.

If going full "lion king" feels too extreme for you, especially when starting out, you can accompany your animal fats and proteins with some dark leafy greens like cooked spinach, and collard greens. The new abundance of healthy fat in your diet will allow you to absorb more nutrients from these veggies than ever before.

Hunter Gatherers:

WE ARE DESIGNED FOR KETO

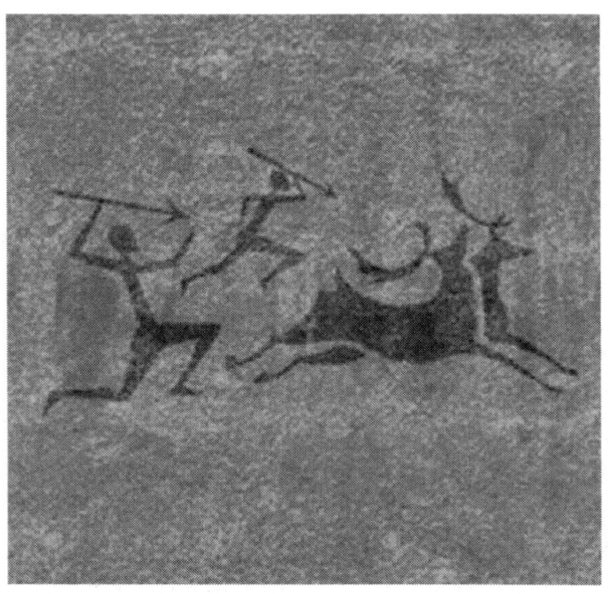

The fact that hikers lost in the woods often survive for weeks without carbohydrates or food of any kind and just water from natural sources is not by chance. It's by design. Our ancestors' DNA was raised on keto, and our DNA is essentially the same as it was 100,000 years ago when humans lived as hunter-gatherers. Way back in the stone age, there were no convenience stores offering processed foods like chips, candy bars, and sodas. Nor were there professional nutritionists admonishing you to eat a so-called "balanced diet" based on grains and vegetables.

Less obvious is the fact that 72% of what we consume today, from processed foods to a wide variety of "natural" foods like fruits, vegetables, nuts, grains, and dairy products, did not exist in the diets of our ancestors.

The early humans you are descended from, and who you are nearly genetically identical to, thrived on a narrow variety of foods and only when their hunting and foraging was successful. When food wasn't available, they fasted until they could find new food sources. Fasting put them into a state of ketosis where their bodies burned stored fat for fuel. Their bodies, and therefore our bodies, are optimized to run without carbohydrates, to go periods without eating, to use fat for fuel, and to thrive on a limited variety of foods.

We don't have to refer back to the fossil record to know this to be true. The living examples of the Hadza and Kung bushmen of Africa who hunt with bows and arrows, get meat on only half their excursions into the savanna in search of wild game. Humans are relatively slow and much weaker than the large prey we once depended on for sustenance. Think of a Woolly Mammoth, other primates, bears, or even herd animals like wildebeests. What allowed us to dominate and multiply was our superior intelligence. Like the bushmen of today, our ancestors made bows and arrows, set traps, and herded animals into optimal hunting zones by strategically setting fires. Trapping, skillfully wielding tools, and cooperating with other humans all require sharp focus and clear, sustained mental energy. It would have been impossible for a glucose-starved brain to take down a mammoth. That's where ketosis comes in. The early humans who couldn't go into ketosis, whose brains and bodies were not able to use fat for fuel, had their genetics literally, and figuratively, stomped out.

WE'RE ALL MEATHEADS

Many scientists believe that the meat, i.e. fat, centered diet of our ancestors was crucial to the evolution of our larger brains.

About two million years ago, we evolved hunting techniques that allowed us to capture and eat calorie-dense animal fat, protein, organs and marrow instead of the low-quality plant diet of apes. This allowed Homo Erectus to take in a surplus of energy at each meal compared to our direct ancestors, the apes. Extra energy in the form of animal fat and protein meant our bodies had the fuel to create bigger brains. This higher quality fuel allowed us to eat less plant fiber which is bulkier than meat, leading us to evolve smaller guts. With less energy going to our gut for digestion, more energy was free to fuel our brain. The results of this evolutionary split are apparent in the fact that the human brain requires 20 percent of our energy when resting. While an ape's brain requires only 8 percent. The take-away is that the human body and brain has evolved to depend and run optimally on a diet of energy dense food. And there's nothing more energy dense than meat.

Supporting the idea that meat is the cornerstone of the diet humans are most evolved to eat, contemporary research into the two hundred and twenty-nine remaining hunter gatherer tribes show that a low carbohydrate and high fat diet is the most common. A 2011 study by Ströhle and Hahn, found that 9 out of 10 of the diets of hunter-gatherer groups had less than a third of calories coming from carbohydrates. These percentages reflect that most hunter-gatherer societies rely on an animal-based diet. Here I hesitate to write "meat," and chose instead the much more accurate term of "animal" because hunter gatherers favored certain parts of the carcass and often discarded other edible parts of the animal—especially the leanest muscle, what today we'd call the tenderloin.

An example of this selectivity is documented by Weston A. Price, a dentist who travelled the world on a quest to study the diets of non-westernized populations that were far healthier than people from his own society. In his book *Nutrition and Physical Degeneration*, Price observed the following practice among Indians living in the Northern Canadian Rockies:

> I found the Indians putting great emphasis upon the eating of the organs of the animals, including parts of the digestive tract. Much of the muscle meat of the animals was fed to the dogs.... The skeletal remains are found as piles of finely broken bone chips or splinters that have been cracked up to obtain as much as possible of the marrow and nutritive qualities of the bones.

The Indians Price observed threw away the muscle meats most prized in the Standard American Diet, and ate only the organ meats and bones, which are higher in fatty-acids, essential minerals, and vitamins.

Similar observations were made by another early twentieth century scientist interested in the link between diet and health in hunter-gatherer populations. Vilhjalmur Stefansson, a Harvard trained anthropologist, went to live with the Inuit in the Canadian arctic. He was the First white man the Mackenzie River band of Inuit had ever seen, and they taught him to hunt and fish with their traditional techniques. Living exactly as they did, he ate Caribou, salmon, seal, and eggs. 70-80% of his calories came from fat, and 99% of all his calories came from meat. Stefansson describes how when eating Caribou, the Inuit most prized the fat behind the eye and the fatty meat around the head, then the organs including the heart, and kidneys; a caribou kidney is 50% saturated fat. And just as the American Indians, the Inuit cast the tenderloin to their dogs.

A few decades earlier another arctic explorer, Lt. Frederick Schwatka, became similarly acquainted with the hunter-gatherer diet of the Inuit. In 1878, Schwatka's team headed deep into the arctic to investigate what had happened to a party of 129 men who had disappeared in 1849. The investigation lasted two years, during which Schwatka and his men lived with the Inuit. For a while, they subsisted on the "white man's" food they brought with them, including fruit cakes and whiskey. But eventually their supplies ran out, and like Stefansson, they hunted and ate as the Inuit, surviving on an all meat diet of reindeer, seal, and bear.

Schwatka's journals from his expedition leave us with what is perhaps the earliest Western account of what today we commonly referred to as the "keto flu," a period of low energy that takes place as your body switches from burning sugar to burning fat.

> When first thrown wholly upon a diet of reindeer meat, it seems inadequate to properly nourish the system and there is an apparent weakness and inability to perform severe exertive, fatiguing journeys. But this soon passes away in the course of two or three weeks... However, seal meat which is far more disagreeable with its fishy odor, and bear meat with its strong flavor, seems to have no such temporary debilitating effect upon the economy.

Schwatka's entry describes the difference between a low-to-no carb diet and a keto diet. When he and his men ate lean reindeer meat, the period of adaptation to ketosis was long and difficult. But when they ate the much fattier bear and seal, their body was fueled with ketones from the outset.

Though Schwatka's experiences of an arctic keto diet were hidden in his journal and not discovered until long after his death, Stefansson returned from his arctic adventure as a very boisterous champion of an all meat, mostly fat, diet. In 1906, well before the mainstream American medical establishment had recommended against meat and demonized fat, Stefansson was met with disbelief verging on antipathy. Some of the fears centered on how an all meat diet could not provide vitamin C, since the vitamin doesn't exist in cooked muscle meat. Doctors assumed a vitamin C deficit would lead to scurvy as it had for many fur trappers and frontiersmen who relied on all meat diets for extended periods.

To prove his detractors wrong, Stefansson and a friend vowed to eat nothing but meat and water for a year. Under the observation of experts from New York's Bellevue hospital, Stefansson and his friend fell ill only once during the entire year, and only after experimenters encouraged them to eat only lean meat. Stefansson describes the experience as inflicting, "dioreah and a feeling of general baffling discomfort." This condition has since been dubbed 'rabbit starvation.' It occurs in diets low in fat and carbohydrates, and high in protein. To this day, military survival manuals warn against eating rabbit if you find yourself in a situation where you have to subsist by hunting and gathering. This condition is due to the inability of the human liver to upregulate urea synthesis to process excessive loads of protein, leading to a whole host of problems including hyperaminoacidemia, hyperammonemia, hyperinsulinemia, nausea, diarrhea, and even death within two to three weeks. Not to fear, Stefansson and friend were quickly cured by a single fat loaded meal of sirloin steak and brains fried in bacon fat.

After the incident of 'rabbit starvation,' experimenters found the ideal ratio to be 3 parts fat to 1-part lean meat, which is, not surprisingly, the foundation of a ketogenetic diet. Furthermore, the fears of scurvy and other nutrient deficiencies never materialized. Stefansson and friend's sterling bill of health is likely because the men ate the whole animal, bones, liver and brains, a practice that is consistent with the diet of the earliest humans.

Raymond Dart, the man who discovered the fossil of our first human ancestor in Africa, describes the earliest humans as, "carnivorous creatures, that seized living quarries by violence, battered them to death... slaking their ravenous thirst with the hot blood of victims and greedily devouring livid writhing flesh." Though his description is a little over-the-top, it conveys the truth of our dietary origins: We came out of the trees not to eat the grass, but to eat the grass eaters!

Our ancestors ate as other large meat-eating mammals do. For instance, our fellow kings of the jungle—lions and tigers—first devour the blood, hearts, kidneys, livers, and brains of their kills, leaving much of the lean muscle to the vultures.

Vestiges of Dart's description of the eating habits of the earliest humans in Africa exist to this day in numerous tribes throughout the continent, including the Masai, whose men eat nothing but meat—often three to five pounds each during celebratory meals—blood, and half a gallon of full fat milk from their Zebu cattle—the equivalent of a half-pound of butterfat. Likewise, the Samburu people eat on average a pound of meat and drink almost two gallons of raw milk each day during most of the year—equivalent to one pound of butterfat. While shepherds in Somalia consume a gallon and a half of camel's milk each day, also equivalent to a pound of butter fat. Each of these tribes get more than sixty percent of their energy from animal fat, yet their mean cholesterol is only about 150 mg/dl (3.8 meq/l), far lower than the average Western person.

In the 1960s prominent doctor and professor George V. Mann, studied the Masai as an example of a population that thrived on a high-fat, low carb, and no vegetable diet. Mann's life work was aimed at confronting what he called the "heart mafia," by which he meant a group of influential figures and institutions in the American medical establishment who built their careers creating and defending erroneous links between the consumption of dietary fat, high cholesterol, and an increase in heart disease. Mann found that despite the Masai's high fat diet, their blood pressure and weight were about 50% less than an average American, and that they experienced almost no heart disease, cancer, or diabetes—the so-called diseases of civilization.

Mann's detractors asserted that African tribes like the Masai were genetically adapted to a high-fat diet. However, a study of Masai people who lived in the Nairobi metropolis showed this to be false. The Nairobi Masai ate considerably less fat, which would suggest to researches taking the genetic inheritance perspective, that their cholesterol should be even lower than their brethren still living in the countryside. Yet the mean cholesterol of the Nairobi Masai was 25 percent higher.

What's more surprising is that the markers of physical health and absence of disease that Mann found in the rural Masai, persisted into old age. These findings fly in the face of the prevailing wisdom of the Western medical establishment that as humans age, cholesterol and weight, along with instances of heart disease, diabetes, and cancer, all inevitably increase.

Mann was not alone in his findings. His work with the aging Masai reflects the earlier observations of Ales Hrdlicka, a doctor and anthropologist, who between 1898 and 1905 surveyed the health of Native American populations in the American Southwest, which he compiled into a 460-page report of the Smithsonian Institute. Studying Native American elders who had lived most of their lives on a diet based on meat from wild game, especially buffalo, before their traditional ways of life were destroyed, Hrdlicka found the population to be in incredibly good health. Malignant diseases were extremely rare, as was dementia and heart disease, of which he found only 3 cases out of the 2,000 people he surveyed. He also found that there were many more centenarians among the Native Americans (224 per million men, and 254 per million women) compared to the whites (3 per million men, and 6 per million women).

Stefansson, Mann, and Hrdlicka's observations of hunter-gatherer and non-western populations thriving on diets based on animal fats are only a few examples among many from our anthropological record. These findings beg the question of whether agriculture was a true step forward for human health? And the answer appears to be a resounding No!

In leaving behind our hunter-gatherer ways of life and diets, we became dependent on crops, mostly grains. Our diets became far less nutritious and diverse. Subsisting on the same grain, i.e. carbohydrates, day in and day out, led to a huge uptick in cavities and periodontal disease that we don't find in hunter-gatherers. Tending to crops all day was more laborious and time consuming than hunting and foraging. Yet this surplus of calories from grain caused populations to boom creating more mouths to feed. And when disease struck or a crop failed, huge portions of the population were afflicted. Suffering from iron, fat, and protein deficiencies, people shrunk, both in terms of their brain size and physical stature.

A S.A.D. LEGACY

"It is not as if farming brought a great improvement in living standards either. A typical hunter-gatherer enjoyed a more varied diet and consumed more protein and calories than settled people, and took in five times as much vitamin C as the average person today."
-Bill Bryson

Today we see the sad legacy of our dependence on agriculture and a diet dominated by carbohydrates. It's ensconced in the misconceived recommendations of the mainstream medical establishment, and it's trumpeted by supposed food gurus like Michael Pollan, whose infamous statement, "Eat food. Not too much. Mostly plants," encompasses everything that's wrong with the way we eat. My rallying cry, which is the same as the vast majority of our human ancestors, is the exact opposite: *Eat fat. Not too little. Mostly from animals!*

Yet we find ourselves in this predicament where study after study is bearing out the same sad story that I've witnessed first-hand as a medical professional for decades: inflammation and stress related diseases like PCOS, diabetes, heart disease, mental disorders, asthma, and autoimmune diseases like IB and ulcerated colitis are skyrocketing among both young and old populations. This increase is a direct result of our modern diets and lifestyles. One recent major study found that more than 75% of people do not meet the minimum requirement of necessary daily physical activity, 72% of modern food types are new in human evolution.

Psycho-emotional stress has increased and is rising dramatically. People are exposed to an overwhelming amount of information on a daily basis. Our genes and physiology, which are almost identical to those of our hunter-gatherer ancestors of 100,000 years ago, preserve core regulation and recovery processes. Yet nowadays, our genes operate in internal and external environments that are completely different from those for which we were designed.

Of course, we cannot go back to our hunter gatherer lifestyle, but we can bring into our modern lives the wisdom of how humans evolved to live. I look at this as the zoo keeper paradox:

A zookeeper's job is to ask if their animals are well adapted to the food and environment that is artificially provided for them. We are human animals. Our modern lifestyles and diets are artificial compared to the world we evolved in for hundreds of thousands of years. In a way we are our own zookeepers. Looking at the historical evidence alongside contemporary medical studies would tell us that we're doing a terrible job of caring for ourselves.

By travelling back in time to gather the wisdom of evolution, my keto way of life is here today to help you care for yourself and improve your fertility, beginning with the food we eat and extending on through to the practices we do to take care of our bodies, minds, and hearts.

INTERMITTENT FEASTING

"Everyone can perform magic, everyone can reach his goals, if he is able to think, if he is able to wait, *if he is able to fast.*"
— Hermann Hesse, Siddhartha

THIS CHAPTER MIGHT JUST SAVE YOUR LIFE

If you're like me and most people I know, you've probably said to yourself something like, Wow it feels good to be hungry before I eat. Maybe you have to go back to a time when you were a kid and you were called inside to dinner after playing for hours with your friends. Or maybe it's something you've felt more recently, perhaps after a hike or a bike ride.

On the flip-side, you've also probably said something like, Wow, I feel like crap. Maybe it was that bag of chips? Or could it have been those granola bars, or that bran muffin? But all I had was oatmeal for breakfast, and a chicken salad for lunch, and stir-fried veggies with rice for dinner, which are all healthy. So why do I feel bloated, tired, and hungry? I bet you've said this more often and more recently than you'd like to admit.

By recalling these two scenarios, we're checking in with our intuitive nutritional intelligence, or in other words, we're listening to our bodies. In the first case, what your body is telling you is that it is designed to be moderately hungry before being fed. In the second case, your body is telling you that it's not designed to eat 3-5 meals a day of grains, lean-proteins, and fibrous, carb-heavy snacks.

If you've never felt either of the above scenarios, you don't know what it's like to be pleasantly hungry before eating, and you're not aware of how your standard American diet is making you sick, it's likely that you've become totally inured to the damage being wreaked upon your body by eating simple carbs all day long. If option three is the case, *this chapter might just save your life!*

Intermittent Feasting

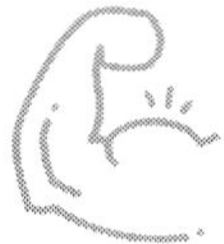

We evolved eating lots of nutrient & calorie dense food in one meal, keeping us full for long

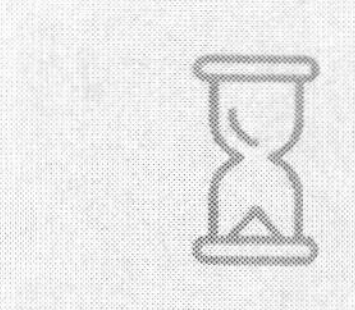

14-16 hours fast to improve overall health and longevity

Get your body burning more fat and less reliant on sugar

The constant intake of abrasive, sugary, food i.e. grazing like a cow, creates a slurry of crap that ferments in your bowels, sending oxidative molecules through your bloodstream to every part of your body. The result is chronic inflammation—the root of nearly all our most prevalent modern diseases including heart disease, diabetes, and cancer.

Yet the mainstream nutritional establishment tells us that we should be eating three meals a day; we should have "healthy" snacks whenever we feel hungry; and that breakfast is the most important meal and should never be skipped. So, it's no surprise that it wasn't until recently that a brave and growing body of researchers, doctors, and nutritionists began to challenge this mainstream dogma with an alternative eating plan called "intermittent fasting," or IF.

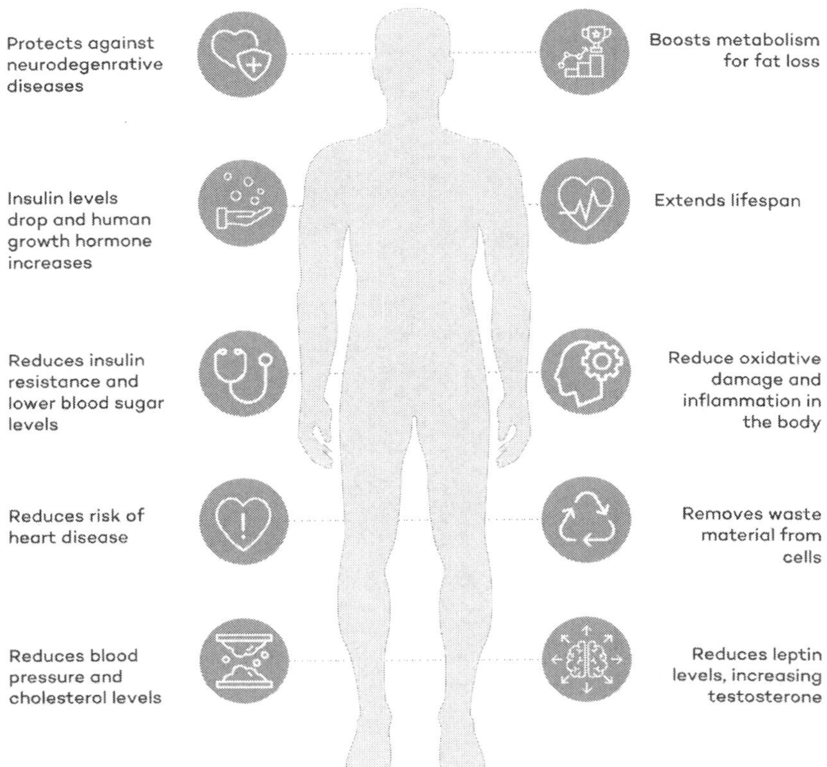
10 Benefits of Intermittent Feasting
Protects against neurodegenrative diseases
Boosts metabolism for fat loss
Insulin levels drop and human growth hormone increases
Extends lifespan
Reduces insulin resistance and lower blood sugar levels
Reduce oxidative damage and inflammation in the body
Reduces risk of heart disease
Removes waste material from cells
Reduces blood pressure and cholesterol levels
Reduces leptin levels, increasing testosterone

I.F. CONTRADICTS MAINSTREAM EATING GUIDELINES

Instead of three meals a day with snacks in between, IF means restricting the number of meals you eat to one or two, and the time frame in which you eat them. Just as the keto diet upends the traditional food pyramid, IF is an about-face to mainstream eating guidelines. And as with keto, IF is informed by looking more closely at the eating habits of paleolithic humans.

Let's remember that 100,000 years ago humans did not have access to a constant supply of food. And, of course, none of it was processed, taken apart and put back together like chips, cookies, and anything with vegetable oils and grain flours. Our ancestors ate whole, fresh foods, especially the fatty parts of animals, and occasionally fruits and nuts when in season and readily available.

Though our bodies are designed to be able to survive weeks without food by switching into ketosis and burning stores of body fat for fuel, most hunter gatherer societies fasted only briefly and intermittently. In fact, evidence shows that hunter gatherers experienced significantly less famine than early agricultural societies. Because agricultural societies were sedentary and relied mainly on one or two staple starches and grains, they lost the cultural knowledge of how to hunt and harvest food from the wild. When their crops failed due to drought, pestilence, and blight, people starved. A well-known and tragic example of the susceptibility of agricultural populations was the 1845 potato famine in Ireland. A single fungus destroyed half the crop of potatoes, resulting in the death by starvation of 1,000,000 Irish and the exodus of a million more.

By contrast, most hunter gatherer societies moved throughout large territories where they employed an extensive cultural knowledge of where and how to harvest a variety of wild, nutrient dense, and seasonally available foods. This combination of mobility, skill, and healthy fat-rich food sources made them much more resilient to natural fluctuations in the cycle of available foods, on both a seasonal and daily basis.

WE ARE DESIGNED TO FAST AND FEAST

Since humans have existed as hunter gatherers vastly longer than as agriculturalists, our DNA is nearly identical to the DNA of our hunter gatherer ancestors. This implies that we share the same craving/consumption cycles, which anthropologists call 'immediate return.' Immediate return means that our ancestors consumed their food completely without waiting, storing, or cultivating.

Most early humans lived amidst an abundance of wild game and food sources so there was no need to ration food, nor incentive to figure out how to preserve it. A hunt meant a feast where everything was eaten. Once the food was devoured, they hunted and gathered again. Acquiring food generally took place in the early part of the day, which meant that people didn't eat until later. The time between feasts marked periods of intermittent fasting. With modern day intermittent fasting techniques, we are mimicking this daily schedule by going 16 or 18 hours without food.

Over hundreds of thousands of years of human evolution, the men and women whose brains and bodies functioned the best in fasted states were the best at hunting and gathering food, and therefore the best at surviving and reproducing. We know that fasting puts the body into ketosis. It follows that ketosis is an optimal metabolic state. It comes as no surprise then that recent studies suggest fasting cycles that induce ketosis followed by recovery periods of feasting, resting, and sleeping, may optimize brain function and resilience, improving mood, energy, and cognition, while increasing resistance to injury and disease.

Yet the same 'immediate return' behavior that benefitted our ancestors during cycles of intermittent fasting becomes a devastating liability in the modern world where we have unfettered access to calorically dense, toxically processed, carb-heavy foods.

For Americans running on a standard carb-based diet (everyone not on keto), abstaining from food for extended periods of time is hard to fathom and even more difficult to put into practice. This is because when you're on a carb-based diet, your body is constantly turning the carbs you eat into blood sugar. This sugar feeds your cells and gives you energy. But carbohydrates are expended quickly so your body is constantly crying out to be refueled. If you're fasting on a carb-based diet, you'll struggle with cravings, lack of focus, low energy, and irritability. When you feast, you'll likely want to binge on a ton of carb heavy foods, spiking your blood sugar, causing fatigue and lack of focus. You'll be stuck on the low to high blood sugar seesaw.

Whereas on a keto diet rich in healthy saturated fats, like our ancestors enjoyed, it can be much easier—and effortless after a little practice—to go twelve, sixteen, and twenty-four hours between feasting.

IF + KETO: A POWERFUL 1-2 PUNCH

When your body is using fat as its primary fuel source, most of your cells get their energy from ketones rather than glucose (sugar/carbohydrates). Fat digests much more slowly than carbohydrates, and ketones pack more energy per unit than glucose, providing your body with a sustained and superior fuel source. Your few cell types that can't use ketones are fed by glucose that is created on-demand in your liver. This means that when you are on keto, your blood sugar never drops to a point where you get hunger cravings and never spikes to a point where you lose focus. Ketones are also effective at suppressing ghrelin, the hormone that makes you feel hungry. In this way, practicing IF on keto increases your ability to lose weight by burning fat for fuel, while allowing you to spend more time not eating. Keto and IF are a one-two punch. But weight loss is only one, and from my perspective, relatively superficial benefit of the radical health transformation that IF+keto initiates within your body. The profound benefits of IF+keto include:

- **Reduced inflammation:** Intermittent fasting reduces oxidative stress and body-wide inflammation markers. This is essential to your health, as recent studies suggest, inflammation is intimately linked with a broad range of non-infectious diseases, perhaps even all of them! In a now famous study of people practicing traditional intermittent fasting for the month of Ramadan, subjects showed significant decreases in proinflammatory and tumor causing molecules called cytokines, as well as decreases in blood pressure, body fat percentage, and body weight.[i]

- **Boosts Human Growth Hormone**: A recent study of 200 participants showed that fasting for a single twenty-four-hour period increased HGH by 2000% for men, and 1300% in women.[ii] HGH is essential for building, maintaining, and repairing healthy tissue in the brain, bones, and other organs, while speeding up healing after injury and repairing muscle tissue after exercise. HGH builds muscle mass, boosts metabolism, and burns fat. Because HGH naturally drops as you age, it becomes even more important to take dietary steps to maintain and increase your HGH levels. HGH has been shown to slow down the ageing process of the skin, reducing sagging and wrinkles.

- **Increases stem cell production**: When you fast, you are essentially resetting your immune system by allowing your body to switch into repair mode. Stem cells increase because they are the primary repair system in your body. They work by morphing into many different types of cells, depending on which parts of your body needs repair. Fasting has been shown to increase stem cells in the intestines, muscles, and brain, while preserving the long-term ability for stem cells to regenerate on their own. The way this works is pretty amazing. When fasting, our bodies greatly reduce our energy expenditure by rapidly shrinking tissues, organs, and populations of different cells in your blood including a whopping 28% decrease in white blood cells. When we enjoy a ***keto feast*** at the end of a fasted period, we are fertilizing this vast crop of new cells the healthiest, most potent food possible. When we combine IF with keto, we're getting rid of tons of damaged cells—especially those damaged from the bonding of sugar molecules in the destructive process called glycation—while our bodies erupt with fresh, fat fueled cells! Lab tests on mice have shown fasting to result in major reductions in the incidence of lymphomas and tumors. The mechanism at work here is the decrease in glucose and insulin—if you're not eating sugar, your body isn't producing insulin. Fasting along with keto starves cancer cells that rely on sugar, while promoting short term atrophy and cell death in a wide range of tissues and organs including the liver and kidneys. Atrophy and cell death here are a good thing because they trigger a period of cellular growth and proliferation driven in part by replenishment during refeeding. But, and this is a big BUT, if you eat sugar and other cancer-causing molecules when feasting at the end of a period of fasting, studies show that you actually increase cancerous activities and pre-cancerous lesions especially in the liver and intestines. This means that keto is not only the best way to get the greatest health benefits out of IF, it's also the best way to protect yourself against the possibility of doing your body harm.

- **Promotes autophagy:** Latin for "self-eating," autophagy is our body's ability to perform its own housekeeping on a cellular level. It's a truly ingenious process where parts of cells called lysosomes dismantle other damaged cell structures such as faulty mitochondria, then re-use these broken parts to generate energy used to create shiny new structures. The exact process is complex, and we're only just beginning to understand it, but already researchers are deeming autophagy a "key in preventing diseases such as cancer, neurodegeneration, cardiomyopathy, diabetes, liver disease, **autoimmune diseases** and infections."[iii] Autophagy is always occurring, but gets what researchers describe as a "profound" boost during fasting. And it has been shown to increase with a keto diet.

- **Increases BDNF, "Miracle-Gro for your brain":** BDNF is short for Brain-Derived Neurotrophic Factor, a naturally occurring growth hormone responsible for neurogenesis—the creation of new neurons. That's why Harvard Neuropsychiatrist, John J. Ratey deemed it, "Miracle-Gro for the brain." Increasing levels of BDNF through intermittent fasting are associated with better moods, higher cognitive ability, more productivity, and better memory while decreasing risks of neurodegenerative diseases like Alzheimer's, dementia, and Parkinson's. Exactly why BDNF gets a boost from fasting isn't totally understood, but I believe it has to do with the way BDNF helps to rapidly form new neural networks. A network is formed when nerve cells in the brain fire together, forming a new thought, memory or skill. We form these networks very quickly in emergency situations when we're kicked into fight of flight mode. When we're fasting, we are in a controlled state of threat. This same healthy dose of stress that stimulates stem cell production, HGH, stem cell production, and autophagy is also the likely the trigger for boosting BDNF.

CHOOSING YOUR PATH

There are a number of popular IF approaches out there to choose from and they all fall into two categories. They are either alternate day fasts, or daily restricted fasts. Alternate day fasting means that you commit to not eating for an entire twenty-four-hour period, usually two days out of each week. This is popularly known as the 5:2 plan.

Daily restricted IF means that you can eat every day, but only within an allotted window of time. I personally practice a daily restricted IF regimen on the narrower end of the spectrum. I eat only one ketogenic meal every twenty-four hours, and I take it in the early evening. I find this gives my body the right amount of time to digest before sleep, while providing the longest period for rest and digestion between meals. I also find that for most people, it's much more difficult to stick with an alternate day plan than it is to simply restrict the time in which you have to eat each day. I know of no evidence to suggest that alternate day fasting is more effective, and my main goal is for you to find an IF practice that's sustainable. For these reasons I recommend, at the very least, to start with a daily restricted regimen.

Everybody is different, and I encourage you to experiment to find what works best for you. Popular daily restricted IF options range from 4, 6, 8, and 10 hours a day where you can eat, while letting your body rest and digest for the remainder of the day. One essential guideline that's important to follow no matter which plan you chose is not to eat late in the evening. Eating later effects your sleeping patterns, and the element of rest is crucial if you are to receive all the benefits of IF outlined above.

14:10 Fasting Clock

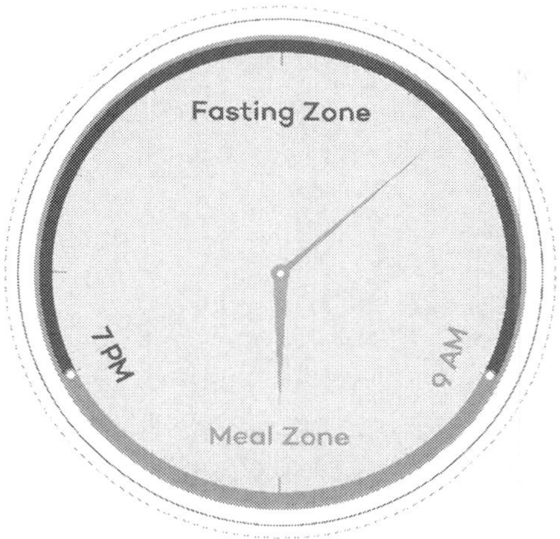

But don't be dismayed, achieving 12-16 hours of IF is much easier than you might think. For instance, if you take your last meal at 7pm, then sleep from 11pm to 7am, and wait to eat until 9am, that's already 14 hours of IF! And if you don't eat until noon, that's 17 hours. As I mentioned earlier, eating a keto diet makes IF so much easier because fat is far more satiating, digests more slowly, and packs more energy than a carb-based diet.

As with all the practices in this book that work together to create my keto way of life, the benefits of IF are profoundly strengthening, and particularly so when practiced in concert with the other tools offered. Skipping breakfast by itself is not going to transform your physique and combat inflammation and disease. You are a mind, body, and soul. Keto is the foundation of bringing the entire picture of you into focus, and IF is here as one of a number of building blocks that you can use to improve your fertility and create the very best version of you!

Beth and Angela's Story

Our daughter was conceived at a fertility clinic in our home state of Michigan back in 2013. Beth was able to conceive relatively easily via IUI with frozen donor sperm, Clomid, and a trigger shot. IUI #4 was a success, and Harper was born at 40+4 weeks in 2014. Within a week of delivering Harper, Beth was rushed back to the hospital and diagnosed with a rare but serious complication of pregnancy called Peripartum Cardiomyopathy (PPCM). PPCM is a form of heart failure that develops during pregnancy, with symptoms presenting around the final months of pregnancy and up to five months postpartum.

Because of this diagnosis and the likelihood of relapsing, Beth was advised against carrying another pregnancy, which at 28 years of age was pretty crushing. Luckily for us, we are a two-mom family and Angela stepped up to the plate. It took about eighteen months for Beth to regain her heart function, and we felt comfortable moving ahead with TTC baby #2.

In February 2016, we scheduled a consult at the clinic where Harper was conceived. At that time, we had 4 vials of our donor sperm in storage and were hoping for another quick and easy conception. Of course, we were wrong. IUI after IUI continued to fail. We used Clomid, Femara, trigger shots, estrogen, progesterone, and nothing was working. After 5 failed IUIs, we decided to move forward with IVF at our clinic in Michigan, partly because it just wasn't working and partly because we were running out of vials of sperm and it was important for our children to have the same donor. The donor actually sold out while we were TTC. Our first round of IVF used our sixth vial of sperm, and we purchased two more as an insurance policy.

The cost of treatment was a huge factor for us, especially after all of the failed IUIs. We have zero insurance coverage for fertility treatments and everything was out of pocket. We regretfully ended up taking out a huge interest personal loan to cover IVF. Allowing our daughter the experience of having a sibling was very important to us, both of us having grown up with siblings of our own.

The more we failed, the more we were driven to succeed. We had our first consult for IVF in August 2016, the same month our daughter turned two. The clinic had us do the Antagonist Protocol for IVF. Angela seemed to be responding well, but slowly, to the medications. In November, Angela had her first egg retrieval. The retrieval was absolutely terrible. None of the nurses on shift could get the IV into her veins. She was stabbed over 4 times in her arms, hands, and wrists. They decided to give up on the IV sedation and just gave her an intramuscular injection of Versed sedation (which did NOT work). She was wide awake for the entire, horrible retrieval.

Regardless, they were able to retrieve 15 eggs, 13 were mature, and 10 were fertilized using ICSI. This clinic believes in two-day transfers, so we returned just two days later for the transfer. We transferred two embryos (their standard practice) and they were able to freeze 4 others. On day 10 we received our beta, which was negative. That first negative from IVF was a blow. We've had many friends succeed their first fresh transfer of IVF at this clinic, and we pretty much assumed this would work for us.

After that was more waiting. The doctors had no explanation for why it failed. This just happens they said. Angela had no known fertility issues, other than a slightly elevated TSH (thyroid) which was managed with medication. For the first FET, we decided to do an endometrial biopsy to check for any infections or endometriosis (and also because they said this would increase our chances for successful implantation). The biopsy was also a really horrible experience, which I will not describe here.

We continued on and scheduled an FET, using the Long Protocol without birth control. Everything looked good, and in February 2017, we transferred two more two-day embryos. On day ten, we got a BFP, but with a low beta (44). We returned every couple days for repeat betas, and the numbers continued to double appropriately. We were over the moon! The second beta was 217. On day 24, she started lightly spotting. The nurses said this could be normal. On day 29, we went for our first ultrasound (6 weeks, 3 days pregnant). The ultrasound technician found the yolk sac, but there was no fetal pole. We were told that the chances of a successful pregnancy were very slim. Another beta draw showed her levels at well over 11,000 and climbing. We were sent home to "wait and see", which is never a fun thing to do.

In week 7, we returned for another scan and there was still no fetal pole, no heartbeat. We were told this was a blighted ovum. We stopped PIO and decided to let the miscarriage happen naturally, which it did. We were told to call the clinic in two weeks if the miscarriage did not happen, but they never told us what to do if it did happen. When we called, they acted as if it was our fault for not contacting them sooner. We were booked for another ultrasound, which happened at the end of May. The scan revealed residual tissue, so Angela required a D&C, which took place in June.

Looking back, we would have done the D&C right away and avoided the trauma that came along with the miscarriage at home. We scheduled another consult, where again they told us there was no explanation, that this just happens sometimes. We got on the schedule for our next (and last) FET using our last two embryos, which took place in August. This time we did an endometrial scratch and sonohistogram prior to transfer. In September, we got the not so unexpected news that this transfer had also failed.

At this point we were hugely in debt, heartbroken, and had nothing to show for it. We scheduled a follow up consult to discuss what happened and where we would go from here, but we ultimately ended up canceling it. We never heard from the clinic again.

We started searching for other fertility clinics in Michigan. There really were no other reasonable options and we couldn't afford another round of IVF at our current clinic. On a whim, Beth posted in a Michigan IVF online group and she was surprised by how many people suggested traveling to New York to visit this clinic called CNY. This seemed totally crazy to me. They described the price and it seemed even crazier! There's no way this could be true. What's the saying, "If something sounds too good to be true, it probably is"? So, we blew this off for a while, but CNY kept popping up in these online forums.

We started researching it. We combed their website and Facebook page, looking for the fine print, looking for the asterisks. We ultimately tried to put this out of our minds because another round of IVF still seemed completely unattainable. In the meantime, we decided to look into foster-to-adopt programs in our area. We went to a foster parent orientation. We ultimately decided this was not the road we wanted to travel for many reasons. The days went on, the seasons turned. In January 2018, we filled out the online request for a consult through CNY's website. Why not, we thought? What did we have to lose?

Turns out CNY is very popular, and we weren't able to get a phone consult until April. We had all of our records faxed over and finally the day arrived. Our phone consult with nurse Catherine Falcon went really well. One look at Angela's records from our fertility clinic and CNY diagnosed her with PCOS, something our fertility clinic never even hinted at. Angela's AMH level was 8.5. They wanted Angela to start taking Metformin. From our research on the CNY Facebook page, we knew that they highly recommended the Keto Diet.

We figured we'd give it a chance, knowing it would help with fertility and also help her PCOS. We ordered The Ketogenic Cookbook and got to work. At the same time, we were searching for a local OB/GYN to do our IVF monitoring for CNY. Keto was quite the adjustment for our carb-loving family, but Angela was committed. She started searching out low-carb alternatives, ditching sugars, and eating lots of bacon.

Our medications arrived in May 2018 and we hurriedly made travel plans for New York. CNY had us on a totally different protocol using low-dose aspirin, low-dose Naltrexone, and prednisone. We were looking at a nearly 9-hour drive and a week-long stay in New York. We were set to arrive the day before Angela's retrieval and leave the same day as the transfer. The results from Keto were almost instant. Angela went on to lose nearly 50 pounds on her Keto journey. We continued to have our follicle monitoring appointments locally until CNY decided it was time to trigger. We triggered in the evening and early the next morning, set out for New York.

At CNY, we were amazed at how warm and welcoming it was. It felt nothing like a doctor's office. Angela's egg retrieval at CNY was WORLDS different from our local clinic. They gave her a soft robe and got the IV in on the first try. She never felt a thing. Angela woke up SMILING, and that was before she even knew that they got TWENTY eggs. 15 of those eggs were mature and 14 fertilized via ICSI. The 14 fertilized eggs turned in to 4 beautiful 5-day blastocysts.

On June 23, 2018, we transferred a gorgeous 4AA blastocyst and the other 3 were put on ice. Angela continued on the Keto Diet throughout our two-week wait and on day 10 we got our BFP! This time we had a strong first beta of 191 which became 432 which became 3,682. At 6 weeks 2 days, we got the first look at our sweet babe with a perfect little heartbeat. Shortly after that scan, we were discharged from CNY to continue care at our local OB/GYN. About a week and a half after CNY discharged us, Angela started to have bleeding. Bright, horrible, heavy bleeding. We thought everything was lost. We mourned yet another loss and failure, after everything we put into this.

At 8 weeks, we had another ultrasound and would you believe it, our little stinker was JUST FINE. They couldn't find any explanation for the bleeding, which continued for several weeks, on and off. Angela is currently 32 weeks pregnant with our son, and we couldn't be more grateful to Dr. Kiltz and the CNY travel team for giving us a second chance. And, because CNY offers in-house financing, we have just about paid off our entire CNY bill, which is a blessing in and of itself, as we will be paying on our first huge interest IVF loan for at least three more years.

INFLAMMATION AND DISEASE

In order to know how and why my keto way of life works to combat disease, increase fertility, and generate well-being that permeates your mind, body, and soul, it is essential that you understand inflammation, its likely causes, and the havoc it wreaks on every organ and system in our bodies.

Inflammation isn't always obvious. It can appear as joint pain or swelling, gum disease, fatigue, headaches, unexplained rashes, and muscle stiffness. Sometimes inflammation goes unnoticed until a diagnosis of heart disease, diabetes, or an autoimmune condition (where the immune system mistakenly attacks your body) such as lupus, multiple sclerosis, and rheumatoid arthritis.

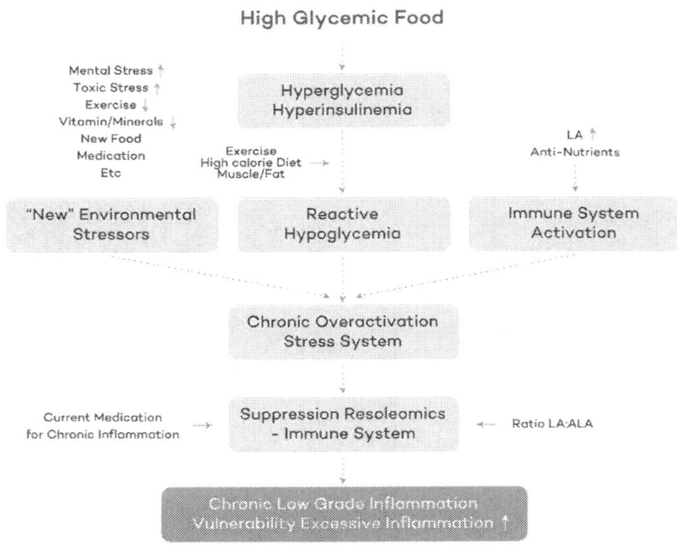

Inflammation is linked to nearly all of our diseases. Infertility is just one among a long list of diseases caused by acute and chronic inflammation due to infection from a microorganism, glucose and glycation, or various phytochemicals and plant antigens—lectins and particles of plant material that elicit inflammatory responses from within our own body.

Pinpointing exactly how inflammation occurs in the uterus, tubes, ovaries or in the male reproductive organs, is still uncertain. But I believe it has to do with blood flow depositing these microorganisms, plant phytochemicals, and antigens into these areas. I also believe that a key contributor to infertility causing inflammation is the excessive heat in the G.I. tract—the colon and small intestines. Fermentation of plant particles (fruits, fibers, vegetables) creates an exothermic reaction that heats and damages local organs and tissues.

TEMPORARY VS. CHRONIC INFLAMMATION

When our body's immune response is functioning properly, inflammation is a temporary response that actually helps the body heal. Inflammation is designed to limit invasions of bacteria and help our cells repair after injury. We evolved inflammation as an essential process for our survival in the absence of modern medication such as antibiotics. But when it doesn't turn off, inflammation simmers at a chronic level, damaging healthy cells instead of healing damaged cells, and contributing to the so-called diseases of civilization, including coronary heart disease, obesity, hypertension, type 2 diabetes, epithelial cell cancers, autoimmune disease, and osteoporosis. The prevalence of these diseases in modern Western society is nothing less than catastrophic.

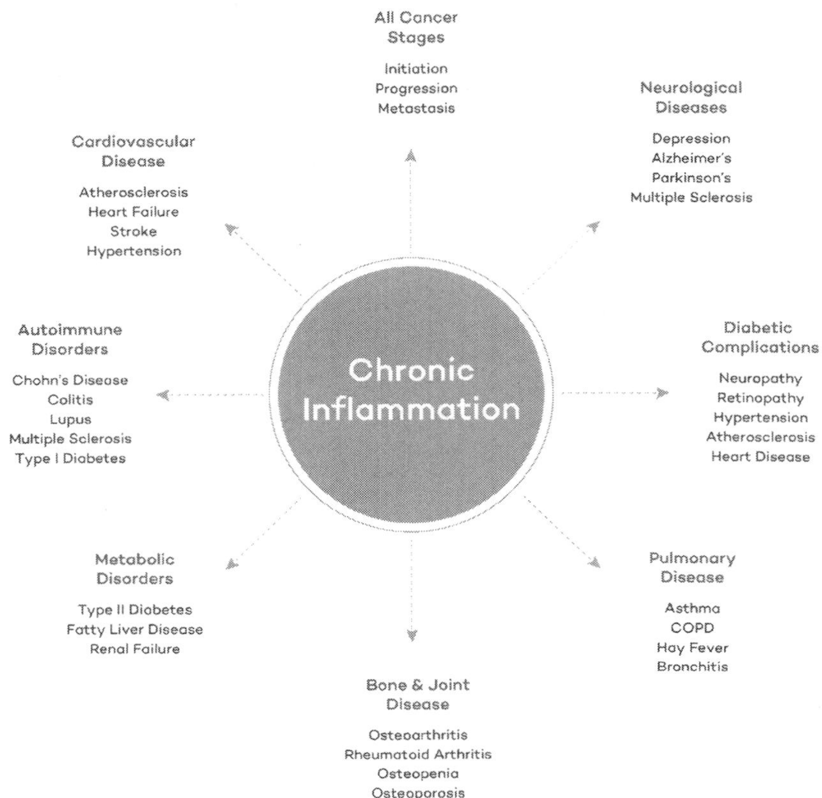

Heart disease is responsible for nearly 25% of the deaths in America. Nearly 75% of American men, more than 60% of women, and nearly 30% of boys and girls under age twenty are either obese or overweight, up from 19% in 1980. 1 out of every 3 adults has hypertension. 10% of the American population has diabetes, while another 70 million Americans are living with pre-diabetes. 38% of American men and women will be diagnosed with cancer in their lifetime. 7% of Americans are living with auto-immune diseases, increasing by over 4% each year, including a 100% increase of Type-1 diabetes between 2001 and 2019. And 50% of Americans aged 50 and older have osteoporosis.

We call these the diseases of civilization because they are virtually non-existent in hunter–gatherers and other non-westernized populations. This point cannot be overemphasized: **The diseases that are killing us by the tens of millions do not exist in societies that live and eat in alignment with their genetic inheritance.**

Remarkably, there are no genetic differences between hunter-gatherer people and modern people that account for their superior health. This tells us that our modern epidemic of chronic inflammation is the result of fundamental changes in diet and lifestyle that occurred after the agricultural revolution around 10,000 years ago, and most dramatically after the Industrial Revolution only 100 years ago.

On an evolutionary time scale, these changes are too recent for the human genome to have adapted. To put this into perspective, during the 10,000 years since the agricultural revolution shifting most of humanity from a diet based on animal fats and proteins to a diet based in carbohydrates from cereal grains, there have only been around 300 generations of humans. That's less than .5% of the history of humans on this planet.

Since the industrial revolution, we have had only 3 generations, yet our modern lifestyles are dramatically different than every generation that has come before us. This rate of lifestyle change is only increasing in our present-day information age, where at the buffet of our all-you-can-eat data plans, we gorge on vastly more information and media—much of it distressing, let alone distracting—than at any previous point in human history. We sleep on average for fewer than 7 hours a night, less than at any previous point in human history, and we consume 12 hours of media, accounting for nearly ¾ of our waking lives.

This all adds up to living in ways that are far more sedentary than we are evolved for. We're saturated with stressful digital information, and we eat a radically different diet where 72% of modern food is new to human evolution, 70% of our nutrient intake is carbohydrates, and 60% of our diet is highly processed foods—foods that have been taken apart and put back together again with various combinations of sugar, corn syrup, salt, oil, preservatives, conditioners and other additives.

We don't have to travel far back in time to see how our modern diet trends track directly with increases in inflammation and disease. Following the recommendations of the mainstream medical establishment since the 1960s, we've had an 8% increase in our consumption of vegetable fats; a 10% decrease in animal fats; a 29% increase in grains; and 17% increase in fruits and vegetables. Yet the entire Westernized population is suffering a global health catastrophe linked to chronic inflammation.

Considering that our natural inflammatory response is designed to produce short, intensive reactions to acute and temporary dangers, the question then becomes, how can we regulate our natural inflammatory response in our fast-changing modern world?

FIVE MAIN CAUSES OF INFLAMMATION & DISEASE

1) **Glucose**
2) **Plant Antigens**
3) **Plant Antinutrients**
4) **Fiber, Bacteria & Yeast**
5) **Exercise**

GLUCOSE

If you're eating the standard American diet, you're consuming 70% carbs, around 20% protein, and 10% fat, including what we mistakenly think of as healthy fats—olive oil, coconut oil, avocado oil. These "vegetable oils" are highly processed products from our industrial food industry, which means we are not evolved to eat them. They are not nearly as healthy and digestible as naturally derived fats like you find marbling the meat of beef, pork, bison, some fish, and wild game. If you're eating the

Standard American Diet, you're sending a steady stream of glucose throughout your whole body, damaging your cells and producing inflammation.

Glucose damages cells through a phenomenon called **glycation**, which is the binding of glucose to every nook and cranny in our bodies, leading to fermentation in the cytoplasm of certain cell lines that can cause tumors and other cancerous cell growth.

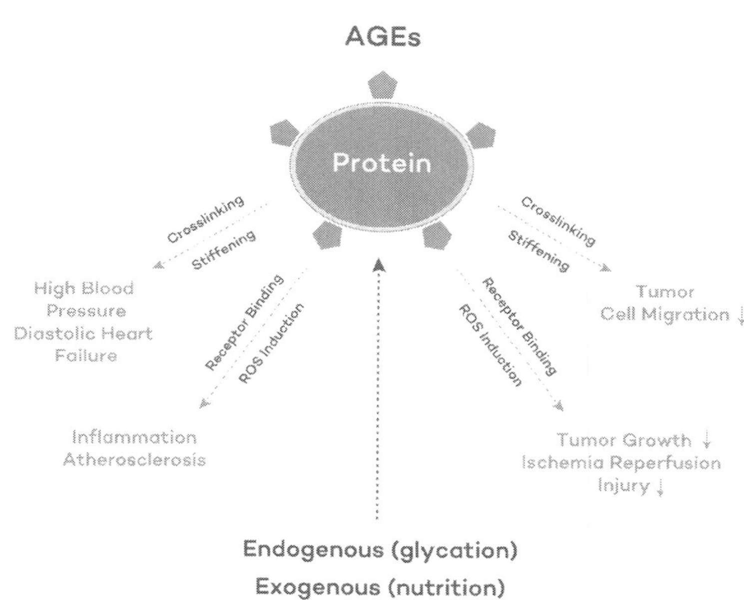

Eating glucose is like carpet bombing your body's cells with sugar. The sugar molecules glom onto your fats and proteins forming what are called "advanced glycation end products," shortened appropriately to AGEs. AGEs cause protein fibers to become stiff and deformed. We've learned most of what we know about glycation by studying diabetics. High blood sugar in diabetics damages connective-tissue and creates chronic inflammation leading to debilitating and deadly conditions such as diseases of the pancreas and liver, cataracts, and Alzheimer's.

In healthy people, glycation causes the same types of cell and tissue damage, only at a more insidious pace. The effects of glycation are most apparent in the aging of skin. Proteins like collagen and elastin that make our complexion springy, plump, and youthful, are extremely susceptible to glycation. When we bomb these proteins with sugars, they become discolored and weak, showing up on the surface of your skin as sagginess, wrinkles, and a dulling of your natural radiance.

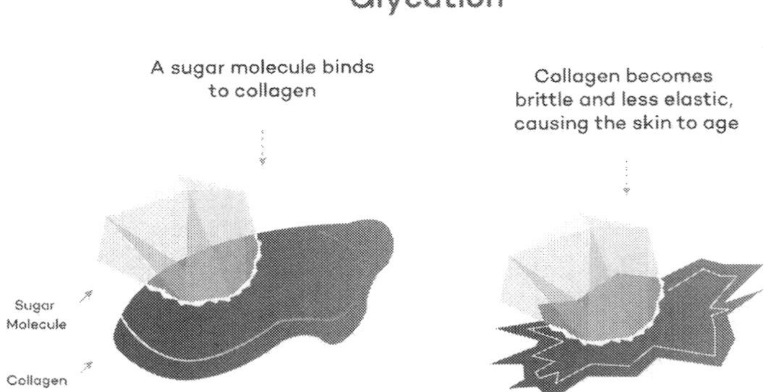
Glycation
A sugar molecule binds to collagen
Collagen becomes brittle and less elastic, causing the skin to age
Sugar Molecule
Collagen

My keto way of life is the most effective defense against creating more glycation, and the best way to get rid of the AGE's that are already in your body. Keto eliminates processed foods along with most refined and unrefined sugars. And when we eat like the kings and queens of the jungle, getting the vast majority of our macronutrient intake from high-quality animal fats and proteins, we are loading our bodies with an incredibly powerful anti-AGE compound called carnosine.

Carnosine is a naturally occurring amino acid that you can only get from your diet by eating meat. It is especially abundant in beef, pork, and turkey breast. Carnosine prevents the cross-linking and stiffening of proteins caused by glycation, which is potent in reducing cognitive decline and Alzheimer's. It also stabilizes atherosclerotic plaques in your blood vessels reducing the risk of stroke and heart attack.

Though all plants are carbohydrates, and all carbohydrates are sugars, white sugar, and high-fructose corn syrup can increase the rate of glycation by 10 times. In addition to these obvious culprits, **AGEs** can be found in many pre-packaged and processed foods that have been preserved, pasteurized, homogenized or refined, such as white flour, cake mixes, dried milk, dried eggs, dairy products including pasteurized milk, and canned or frozen pre-cooked meals. High heat, dry-cooking and browning can also increase AGEs in food. Consider switching to low-heat and moisture intensive techniques like steaming, boiling, poaching, stewing, stir-frying or using a slow cooker.

If you rely on caffeinated beverages to get you through the day, I recommend swapping coffee for green tea or matcha, which has been proven to significantly interfere with the glycation process while stimulating collagen synthesis. Collagen is the most abundant protein in our bodies, and we depend on collagen synthesis to maintain and repair not only our skin, but our bones, ligaments, muscle tissue, and teeth.

FRUITS AND VEGETABLES

Most people think of plant-based food sources as "healthy" carbs. But our body can't tell the difference between a candy bar and an apple. Carbon dioxide from the air, plus sunlight and water form long chain carbohydrates. This is the process of photosynthesis that builds trees, vines, leaves, fruits, and roots. Plant carbs and refined sugars have a very similar chemical makeup and they get processed in the body in the same way. Every carb we eat, from lettuce to a lollipop, is eventually broken down into basic sugar.

This is a simple yet difficult truth for most people to accept. Other than the revelation that high-quality saturated fat is actually good for you, the part of my keto way of life that is particularly surprising to nearly everyone I talk to is my recommendation of eating little to no fruits, vegetables, and fiber.

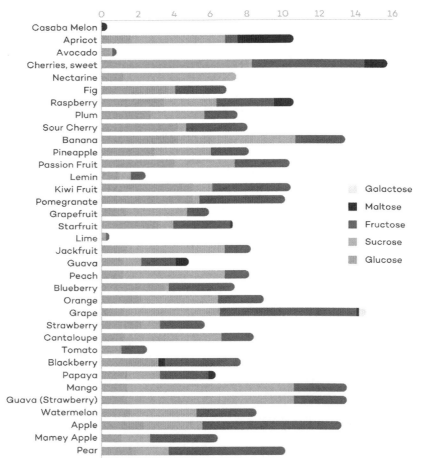

Fruits by percent composition of sugar

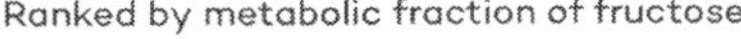

Since you were a kid, you've probably been taught that a big salad is the epitome of health, or how about a plate full of steamed broccoli? For most of you, the idea that you should eat fewer veggies is hard to swallow. But just take a look at the graph revealing the glycemic index on some of your most beloved fruits and vegetables from blueberries to onions—they're loaded with sugar and carbs.

They also contain high amounts of plant antigens, antinutrients, and phytochemicals; molecules that harm our bodies on a cellular level, eliciting immune reactions that lead to chronic disorders and disease.

For instance, many cruciferous vegetables (the *Brassica family),* such as broccoli, cauliflower, cabbage, etc. *that rule the produce section, have a bitter taste, and a sulfurous smell when cooked. Our instinctive response to bitterness and sulfur is to stay away. Just watch what happens when you put a steaming plate of broccoli in front of a young child who hasn't been indoctrinated into the belief that broccoli is good for her.*

Crucifers, like many other plant families, have evolved these repellant characteristics so that we don't want to eat them. Their smell and taste defenses are just the tip of the iceberg. Those chemicals are the first sign of sophisticated natural pesticides created to kill insects, larvae, worms, fungi, and bacteria. A single plant can contain an arsenal of chemical defenses including molecules that recognize invaders, attach to them, and kill them. Poisons that destroy cells and mitochondria by exploding their membranes. Enzyme inhibitors that interfere with vital metabolic reactions, and oxidative toxins that fracture strands of DNA.

Just as animals have evolved camouflage and poisons for protection and perpetuation, plants are equipped with chemicals that both seduce us into eating them and protect them from being digested so that their seeds are spread and fertilized through our waste. These compounds include naturally-occurring pesticides, mineral chelators, and antibiotics. Like humans, plants are evolved to accomplish one goal, and that's to reproduce. Being a healthy food for humans is rarely in a plant's best interest. Plants have been on earth for hundreds of millions of years, humans have been on earth for a mere 500,000 years. Who do you think has the upperhand when it comes to survival?

Let's take broccoli as a case study to get a closer look into the sophisticated defenses hidden within the plants we're told are good for us. Like other cruciferous veggies, broccoli uses chemicals to protect itself, in particular *sulforaphane.* Yet when broccoli is safely soaking up the sun in a field, none of this chemical is present. This is because sulforaphane is so toxic to living cells, including broccoli's own cells, that the two molecules that combine to make it are stored separately within the broccoli. But when broccoli is attacked by insects, animals, or humans by biting into its flesh, the separate compartments are breached and the two molecules—glucosinolate and myrosinase—combine to make sulforaphane, a poisonous pesticide with the power to kill insects, worms, and bacteria.

Sulforaphane works by poisoning mitochondria, inhibiting cellular manufacturing and detoxifying centers, creating free-radical oxidants (the opposite of anti-oxidants) that wreak havoc on our cellular tissue, depleting other crucial antioxidants, and interfering with iodine absorption crucial for thyroid function. These same processes that kill small critters, kill and damage human cells causing inflammation, and in some cases, even cancerous malfunctions.

PLANT ANTIGENS

We are allergic to many plant antigens. Just ask yourself how many people you know who are allergic to various nuts and seeds, sulfuric vegetables, and fruits.? Then ask yourself if you know anyone allergic to fatty meat? Okay, you might know someone who is allergic to some plant that the animal is eating, but it's highly unlikely that anyone is allergic to the meat itself. I'm also not a big believer in all of this turkey and chicken. The process that brings it to market exposes it to too much contact with microorganisms in the air and the environment. It's too lean. All of this lean meat simply converts to fat in the liver.

But my biggest concern is plant antigens. My daughter is allergic to avocados and bananas. I know so many people allergic to strawberries. And kale can be a quiet killer. It's simple. Kale is sugar. It's got all of these antigens that you're allergic to. I know it sounds wild, and I didn't believe it at first either. But every day I'm discovering how powerful the food industry is at convincing us what we should BUY to eat. This is the reason the agricultural industrial food complex recommends so much variety and outlines so many "needs" in the form of specific minerals and vitamins. It's a marketing ploy!

As a physician working directly with bodies every day, witnessing first-hand how a diet with a limited variety of foods and a foundation of high-quality fats improves health and fertility, I honestly can't make heads or tails out of most mainstream diet recommendations.

ANTINUTRIENTS

Antinutrients are natural components of food and especially prevalent in plant foods. They are found in abundance in most of the foods we've been led to believe are healthy, including wholegrains, nuts, legumes, wine, grapes, and chocolate. But when we ingest them regularly, they attack our bodies causing inflammation that leads to infertility and disease.

Phytates, found in whole grains, legumes and nuts, are used by plants to store phosphorous. Yet they don't make it available to our bodies. Instead phytates bind to our own minerals and nutrients, especially calcium, iron, zinc, magnesium, copper and some proteins. Once bound by phytates, these minerals are no longer available to our bodies to use. Nutrient deficiencies caused by phytates are most common in unvaried diets high in cereal grains. The presence of phytates in grains is one of the main factors in the decline in vitality markers including height and bone density, and the rise in disease that occurred during the agricultural revolution when most of the human population switched from a majority meat diet to an almost exclusively grain diet.

Lectins, found in legumes, whole grains and to a lesser degree in dairy, seafood, the nightshade family of vegetables (i.e., tomatoes, peppers, eggplant, potatoes) bind directly to the lining of the small intestine, inhibiting absorption of nutrients and causing lesions on the intestine leading to leaky gut syndrome. They also facilitate the growth of bacteria strains which contribute to endotoxemia, a type of low-grade inflammation that affects approximately 33% of the Western population, and can cause inflammatory bowel disease, ulcerative colitis, and Crohn's disease. Most plant lectins are relatively resistant to heat and digestive enzymes.

Protease Inhibitors, widely distributed within the plant kingdom, including the seeds of most cultivated legumes and cereals. Protease inhibitors are the most commonly encountered antinutrients in plants, and they block the digestive enzymes that break down proteins in our digestive tract.

Saponins, like most other antinutrients, are found primarily in legumes and grains. They're the chemicals that create the foamy substance on the surface of water when you soak beans. Saponins harm us by binding to various nutrients, inhibiting our ability to use them. Saponins inhibit digestive enzymes causing a decrease in protein digestibility and absorption. And some saponins even have the ability to breakdown red blood cells.

FIBER = BACTERIA + YEAST + VIRUSES + MICROORGANISMS

Fibers are complex carbohydrates and strands of poorly or non-digestible carbs that abrade and inflame the bowels. Insoluble fiber is like steel wool in our gastrointestinal tract and sandpaper in the gut. It damages and destroys the very sensitive mucosal lining of the gastrointestinal tract. Soluble fiber from plants ferments in our bodies as it breaks down. When you chew fiber, you simplify it and expose it to bacteria and yeasts that feed on it during the process of digestion. Fermentation of plant materials produces heat, gas, aldehyde, alcohol, and methane. The pressure it creates can lead to hemorrhoids and GERD.

The nutritional-agricultural-industrial-complex recommends that we fill our guts with poorly or non-digestible fiber (carbohydrates) that we get mainly from grains. Hence, the ever-popular raisin bran cereal and bran muffins. Yet when fiber gets down to the colon,

it adds bulk to enlarge the feces making it more difficult to expel through the small exit portal. So why is fiber recommended in the first place?

Fiber has been shown to moderately reduce blood sugar spikes by slowing down the normal process of digestion. However, when you're practicing my keto way of life, there is absolutely no need to protect against blood sugar spikes because you aren't eating any sugar in the first place! Fiber is also recommended because it can reduce LDL cholesterol. But LDL cholesterol ceases to be a problem when we cut out carbs and follow the keto diet. Our liver makes 75% of the cholesterol we need, and it's up to us to get the other 25% from high-quality animal sources.

What about the widespread belief that fiber is good for colon health and that it protects against cancer? It's a total myth. Doctors Tan and Seow-Choen, in the World Journal of Gastroenterology looked at all the studies over the previous 35 years investigating the link between fiber and colon health:

> "A strong case cannot be made for a protective effect of dietary fiber against colorectal polyp or cancer. Neither has fiber been found to be useful in chronic constipation and irritable bowel syndrome. It is also not useful in the treatment of perianal conditions. The fiber deficit-diverticulosis theory should also be challenged... we often choose to believe a lie, as a lie repeated often enough by enough people becomes accepted as the truth. We urge clinicians to keep an open mind. Myths about fiber must be debunked and truth installed."

The truth is, fiber fuels the fire of inflammation. Bacteria and yeast ferment fiber to make heat, alcohol, and aldehydes that fuel the inflammatory processes in the body leading to colitis, irritable bowel, Crohn's, hemorrhoids, you name it. Alcohol in the colon, rectum, and the digestive tract, travels to millions of cells throughout our bodies damaging them as if we were drinking alcohol. The millions of bowel surgeries and bowel problems people are experiencing as a result are overwhelming. A 2005 study shows that 35 out of every 100 Americans visited the hospital for bowel related ailments.

I myself was so indoctrinated into the belief that fiber was essential to health that I didn't trust this counter-narrative until I eliminated fruits and vegetables, and my digestion became the best it's ever been. Our bodies are finely tuned to nurture and heal themselves if we feed them the right food. But we can't heal if we're constantly filling our bodies with inflammatory products (alcohol, fruits, fibers, vegetable) and not enough fat.

MY BEEF WITH VEGGIE STUDIES

Before moving on to non-diet related causes of inflammation, I want to briefly discuss how I came to my realization that vegetables are not necessary, nor proven to be healthy. And in many cases, unhealthy, despite the so-called scientific evidence.

I've poured over hundreds of studies, and I haven't come across a single one that pits veggie eaters head-to-head against non-veggie eaters. Most of these studies either lump fruits and vegetables together or test for the benefits of highly concentrated plant extracts. None of them control for the consumption of complex carbohydrates, and very few take into consideration demographic and lifestyle choices like income, physical activity, and alcohol consumption.

I also find that the vast majority of studies are conducted in order to convince people to eat more vegetables, i.e., to support the researchers' hypothesis, rather than to simply and straightforwardly test veggies for their health benefits. Most of these studies are what we call "epidemiological," which are not true experiments, but rather comparisons where researchers cherry pick data that supports their hypothesis while ignoring more significant variables.

Take for example a study based in Finland and another in Japan, suggesting that people who eat lots of fiber (30-35 grams per day) may reduce their risk of coronary heart disease. These epidemiological studies followed over 22,000 Japanese and 50,000 Finnish people. At the end of the observation, researchers compare the group that ate the most fiber with the group that ate the least, measure the occurrence of disease in each, and make up conclusions about cause and effect connections.

The problem with this kind of study is that fiber consumption—or consumption of any plants in these types of studies—is far from the only factor shared by members of each group. The group that ate more fiber is likely to be more generally health-conscious because they've been brainwashed into thinking fiber is healthy long before the observational period. I'd bet they drink less alcohol, smoke less, and eat less junk food. This means that based on these studies, a cause-and-effect connection between fiber consumption and heart health is bogus.

Not surprisingly, there have been a slew of recent articles revealing the shortcomings of similar studies, including the 2005 article by highly-regarded Stanford physician-scientist, John P. A. Ioannidis, titled, *Why Most Published Research Findings Are False.* One of the key points he makes is that the hotter a scientific field (with more scientific teams involved)—and nothing has been hotter for longer than the attempt by the mainstream medical industry to get us to eat more plants—the less likely the research findings are to be true.

When there are many competing personalities involved, as there are in the nutritional health debate, getting ahead of the competition becomes the top priority and can lead to rushed, shoddy experiments and false correlates. To make my way through all this bad science, I rely on my first-hand observations of thousands of patients, and I've learned to read between the lines of the scientific literature.

For instance, a study from the 2002 *British Journal of Nutrition,* sought to see if green tea anti-oxidants worked. To make sure the effects were from the tea, researchers removed fruits and veggies from the diets of their subjects. Though the green-tea antioxidants showed no long-term effects, the researchers found instead that the removal of the fruits and veggies created a "decrease in protein oxidation ... and an increased resistance of plasma lipoproteins to oxidation." Pointing to a "more general relief of oxidative stress after depletion of flavonoid and ascorbate-rich fruits and vegetables from the diet, contrary to common beliefs." In other words, not eating fruits and vegetables was healthier than eating them.

STRENUOUS EXERCISE: THE HAMPSTER WHEEL OF INFLAMMATION

We've got to move intentionally and regularly to stay healthy, but excessive and high-impact exercise damages our bodies. Strenuous exercise causes heat in the gut and joints. It robs the blood flow from our core and our brains where it's most needed, sending it to the muscles of our extremities. Excessive exercise puts our adrenals into hyper-drive and constricts our blood vessels.

I'm not suggesting you sit still and "veg-out." Intentional movement is essential. I recommend practices like yoga and Tai chi. Keep it relaxed. Go for a hike in the woods and immerse yourself in nature. Walk with a friend to catch up and deeply connect. Be creative with your physical movement. Paint. Do pottery. Sing. Dance. Do something physical that inspires you every day, but stay off the treadmill, the elliptical, the stationary bike, and leave the grueling boot-camp training to the marines.

Again, let's take our cue from the kings and queens of the jungle. Lions don't exercise! Yes, they walk around a bit. They hunt. They feast, feed, and reproduce. This is how animals at the top of the food chain—you and me!—ought to live. Let's acknowledge the fact that we are human animals with simple, natural requirements: eating, drinking water, relaxed movement, and reproducing, all within the security of our herd who we bond with through loving cooperation.

Sugar Isn't Sweet

I believe that sugar is the root cause of infertility along with the chronic diseases most likely to kill us, including heart-disease, diabetes, and cancer. Sugar is responsible for our national health epidemic characterized by startling statistics like the fact that 3 out of 4 Americans are overweight, cardiovascular disease is at an all-time high, and 1 out of 11 *children* suffer from non-alcoholic fatty liver disease.

The average American consumes a staggering 3 pounds of sugar each week, much of it hidden in processed foods. Many "healthy," low-fat food options that we don't consider to be sweet, like tomato sauce and yogurt, are packed with sugar. It's common for food manufacturers to bump up the sugar to maintain flavor and texture when they produce "low-fat" and "non-fat" products. That fancy drink from your coffee shop, or "lite" dressing on that "healthy" salad you had for lunch has way more sugar than you'd expect.

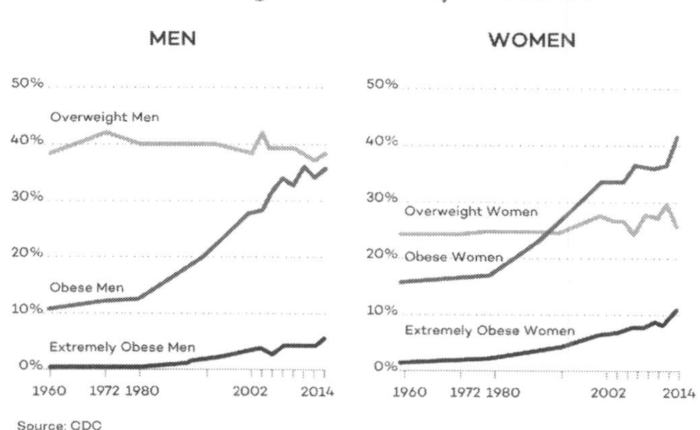

Though sugar is in most of the foods we eat, our body has no need for sugar. Ever. Your liver can make all the glucose it needs from just about anything—protein, fat, or carbs. Contrary to what you might have believed, carbohydrates (sugars) are a non-essential part of our diet. Sugar is a quick energy source and breaks down quickly, but fat is a much better fuel in every way.

Hidden Sugar Content In Everyday Food

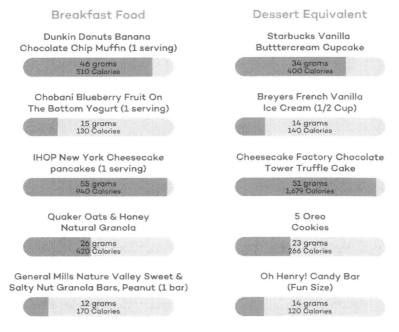

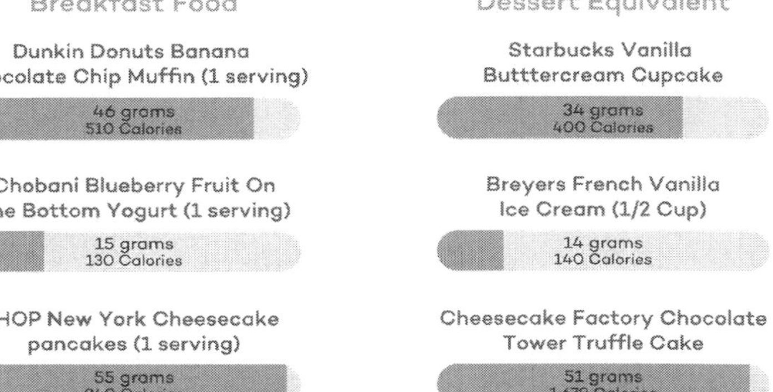

Sugar has the same toxic effect on the liver as alcohol, and it activates the same addictive circuitry of the brain as cocaine and heroin. I know it's hard to hear it, but fruits and vegetables are just sugar too. This is the reason why the dietary recommendations of the American Diabetes Association and the American Heart Association are so frustrating to me. I lost my beautiful sister Maria Ann to diabetes. She was diagnosed at age four and died at 52, blind and from heart disease as a result of diabetes. I now know that the diet recommended to her by her doctors was completely wrong. Sugar comes from all plant material! Eating a diet rich in fresh fruits and vegetables increased her glucose levels, accelerating organ damage and expediting her death.

Every single one of these names on a food label...

Agave juice
Agave nectar
Agave sap
Agave syrup
Beet sugar
Brown rice syrup
Brown sugar
Cane juice
Cane sugar
Clintose
Confectioner's
Powdered Sugar
Confectioner's sugar
Corn sweetener
Corn syrup
Corn glucose syrup
Date sugar
Dri-mol
Dri-sweet
Dried raisin
Sweetener
Edible lactose
Flo-malt

Fructose
Fructose sweetener
Glaze and icing sugar
Glaze icing sugar
Golden syrup
Gomme
Granular sweetener
Granulated sugar
High-fructose corn
Syrup
Honey
Honi-bake
Honi-flake
Inverted sugar
Isoglucose
Isomaltulose
Kona-ame
Lactose
Liquid sweetener
Malt
Malt sweetener
Malt syrup
Malotose

Maple
Maple sugar
Maple syrup
Mizuame
Molasses
Nulomoline
Powdered sugar
Rice syrup
Sorghum
Sorghum syrup
Starch sweetener
Suconat
Sucrose
Sucrovert
Sugar beet
Sugar invert
Sweet 'n' neat
Table sugar
Treacle
Trehalose
Trusweet
Turbinado sugar
Versatose

= Added Sugar

SOURCE: The Lancet: "Sweetening of the global diet, particulary beverages: patterns, trends, and policy responsees" Barry M. Popkin. Corinna Hawkes, 2015

Sugar goes by over 60 different names: glucose, fructose, sucrose, maltose—to list a few. But our body processes them all the same way by sending a portion of these sugars through our blood stream, while sending the excess to the liver to be converted into fat. Although we're told that lettuce, for example, is a "complex" carb, it's really full-on glucose, just as every plant material we consume is also sugar. Our body processes lettuce similarly to how it processes table sugar. Most fruits contain fructose—also a simple sugar like the glucose in lettuce. We don't need any of it, and it's certainly not the optimal fuel for the body and mind

Here are some things I've learned about sugar and our diets:

- **Sugar is addictive.** When we eat sugar, we activate opiate and dopamine receptors in our brains. Ironically, these are the same "happy" chemicals that cause us to feel good when hanging out with loved ones and good friends. But with sugar we get stuck in a compulsive loop of consumption despite the negative consequences like weight gain, hormone imbalances, and inflammation leading to cancer and other chronic and degenerative diseases. Studies suggest that every time we eat sweets, we are reinforcing the neuropathways associated with addiction, causing the brain to become increasingly hardwired to crave sugar. The more sugar we eat, the more tolerance we build up, the more sugar we need to get our fix, the worse it is for our body and brains. Speaking of our brains, diets high in sugar reduce the production of BDFN, a key growth hormone in the brain that protects us against age-related neurodegenerative diseases. By contrast, a keto diet increases the production of BDFN.

Sugar creates an unhealthy addictive cycle like any other drug, and in fact researchers in France have determined that the rewards experienced by the brain after consuming sugar are even "more rewarding and attractive" than the effects of cocaine.[iv] Indeed, research on rats from Connecticut College has shown that Oreo cookies activate more neurons in the brain's pleasure center than cocaine (and yes, the rats would eat the filling first just like humans).[v]

- **Sugar causes cancer**: A 2019 study links drinking just a small 100 ml glass of a sugary drink per day, which is only a third of a typical can of soda, to an 18% increase in overall cancer risk and a 22% increase in risk for breast cancer. Not surprisingly the increased risk of cancer in consuming sugary drinks was observed even among consumers of pure fruit juice. Mathilde Touvier, the research director of the Nutritional Epidemiology Research Team of the National Health and Medical Research Institute at the Paris 13 University, states, "What we observed was that the main driver of the association seems to be really the sugar contained in these sugary drinks." These warnings about the dangers of sugar drinks are especially potent in light of the fact that about half of the sugar the average American consumes comes from soda and fruit drinks, which, not surprisingly, are the number one source of hollow-calories (those without any nutritional benefit) in our diet.

The cells of many human cancers depend on blood sugar to grow and multiply, and even develop mutations that allow them to increase the energy they get from insulin. Researchers believe that many pre-cancerous cells would never become malignant tumors if they weren't being fueled by sugar.

- **Sugar causes metabolic syndrome:** Chances are you've never heard of metabolic syndrome, but it's a huge problem afflicting over 70 million Americans, so there's a good chance you have it! The most obvious sign of metabolic syndrome is simply being overweight. And it's most likely you're overweight because you eat a lot of sugar and carbs. When you eat sugar, your body secretes insulin to process the sugar and keep your blood sugar levels in control. Metabolic syndrome occurs when you eat too much sugar to the point where your cells become resistant to insulin. Your pancreas responds to rising blood sugar by dumping more and more insulin into your bloodstream. This exhausts the pancreas, and when the pancreas craps out, your blood sugar balloons out of control, i.e. you've got diabetes. Yet even before full blown diabetes, the excess insulin that occurs with metabolic disease results in higher triglyceride levels and blood pressure, increasing your body's resistance to insulin and increasing your risk of a heart attack. This whole cycle is what we call metabolic syndrome, and you have sugar to thank for it.

- **There is nothing better or worse about High Fructose Corn Syrup than normal table sugar**. Just because something says, "No High Fructose Corn Syrup," does not mean it's any less lethal than standard refined sugar. This kind of labeling is a marketing scam. Both sugars are deadly because each ends up as glucose and fructose in our guts. Our bodies react the same way to both, and their effects on our bodies are the same.

- **Artificial sweeteners are no alternative:** A recent study found that drinking two or more of any kind of artificially sweetened drink a day was linked to an increased risk of clot-based strokes, heart attacks and early death in women over 50.[vi] Sweeteners activate the same neural reward pathways as sugar! When we eat artificial sweeteners, we're screwing with our bodies natural reward centers. We eat and crave sweet things because sweet foods in the natural environment usually mean loads of quick calories. Yet alternative sweeteners give us incomplete satisfaction by sending mixed signals through our metabolic system. The first signal is that we have eaten something sweet, then the second is that we haven't actually consumed the calories associated with the sweetness. Our bodies respond by seeking more calories. Common artificial sweeteners including aspartame, sucralose, or saccharin, cause insulin resistance by fertilizing toxic gut bacteria (Firmicutes). This bacteria takes energy from our food and stores it as fat. After a 5-day research period where participants were fed the FDA's maximum dose of saccharine, 60% developed glucose intolerance.

WHAT IS INFERTILITY?

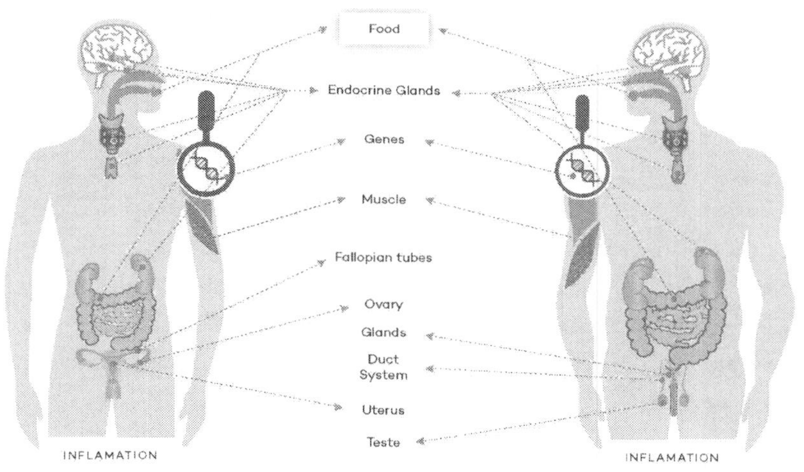

Infertility is most often defined as the inability to conceive after 12 months of regular unprotected intercourse. However, I've seen many factors including age, medical history, and testing that can lead to a clinical diagnosis of infertility long before a year of trying to get pregnant. Infertility affects approximately 1/8 of the population. It doesn't discriminate across any demographic or ethnic boundary and has many potential causes. But I believe that a ketogenic diet and a lifestyle that supports your whole self, mind, body, and spirit is the most powerful treatment for infertility.

The key to keto's effects on fertility is in how keto reduces insulin levels in both men and women. Reducing insulin allows the body to rebalance sex hormones. Healthy hormone cycles are crucial to fertility by allowing women to resume regular ovulation and increasing sperm counts in men.

The science supporting the link between insulin and infertility is alarmingly clear. A 2012 study showed that as carb intake increased in men, sperm counts declined. And a large-scale 2009 study by the Harvard School of Public Health that followed 18,555 women with no history of infertility over eight years, discovered that among the 438 women who reported infertility, there was a correlation between high sugar and carb intake and their difficulty getting pregnant.

I've seen countless patients who consider keto a miracle. But from my perspective, it's common sense. Less sugar means less insulin. Less insulin allows your hormones to balance while decreasing inflammation in your reproductive organs. Healthy cycles, healthy sperm, and healthy tubes will give you your best chance at pregnancy, while saving you stress, time, and money on all the pricks, pokes, and procedures of mainstream fertility treatments.

Once keto helps you successfully conceive, it's important that you consult with your doctor to make sure you are receiving a full range of nutrition for you and your baby. Supplements of folic acid and potassium may be necessary, and you may need to add in more carbohydrates and potassium from healthy sources like bananas and some legumes along with folate-rich foods like dark leafy greens. It's important to remember that every body, and every pregnancy is different and may require specific nutrients accordingly.

Keto for PCOS

As a fertility doctor, PCOS is one of the first disorders I look for when patients come to me for help. So, before we get into just how and why keto treats PCOS, let's take a look at how PCOS can show up in your life.

Do you have trouble knowing when and if your period is on its way? Do you go months without having your period? Do you have abnormal hair growth on places like your face, chest, tummy, fingers, and toes? Is your hair thinning? Do you have acne? Does maintaining a healthy weight feel like a never-ending battle against your own body? Do you have skin tags or dark spots in the folds of your armpits and neck? Are these physical symptoms coupled with fatigue, low sex drive, mood swings, depression or anxiety?

If any or all of these difficult and embarrassing symptoms sound familiar, you may have Polycystic Ovarian Syndrome.

PCOS is the most common cause of infertility in women, and it affects between 10 and 18% of women of childbearing age. Yet, because it's rarely diagnosed until later in life when women are trying to get pregnant, less than half of women with PCOS know they have it. That means millions of women are living with PCOS, and likely suffering from infertility, without knowing why. Thousands of patients with PCOS have come through the doors of my clinics, and after helping these same patients successfully conceive and give birth, I've discovered that the most effective treatment I can recommend is a keto way of life.

To understand why keto cures PCOS, let's look at exactly what a cyst is and why it impedes fertility. Quite simply, a cyst is a fluid-filled sac. Cysts can occur anywhere in the body. Women with PCOS develop cysts on their ovaries when, over time, eggs are not being released properly. This is why PCOS corresponds with an irregular menstrual cycle.

Normally, you're supposed to get your period about every twenty-eight days when your ovaries release an egg to get fertilized. As the egg matures, a sac forms around it on the surface of your ovary. Then the egg and the sac are released together into your uterus. If the egg is fertilized by a lucky sperm, you're pregnant. If it is not fertilized, the uterus sheds the egg along with the preemptive womb lining, i.e., you get your period.

But when you have PCOS, either the egg remains attached to the surface of your ovary where it continues to grow, or it's released but it leaves the sac behind. The remaining sac can reseal and fill with fluid causing a cyst. Over time, you can see the build-up of these cysts with an ultrasound. Doctors often refer to them as a "string of pearls."

These egg release malfunctions are caused by a hormonal imbalance where too much luteinizing hormone (LH) and not enough follicle-stimulating hormone (FSH) are produced in your body. High levels of LH cause your body to produce androgens, which are male hormones such as testosterone. You don't need a medical degree to make the connection between high levels of male hormones and problems with female reproductive processes.

As with most diseases and disorders, mainstream medicine still doesn't know exactly what causes PCOS. The official position is that PCOS, like almost everything that has to do with our health, is due to a combination of genetic and environmental factors—telling us pretty much nothing. Unsurprisingly, there's no known cure, only medications that can temporarily treat some of the symptoms.

What we do know about PCOS is that it is strongly correlated with obesity, defects in insulin secretion, insulin resistance, and inflammation that causes polycystic ovaries to produce excess male hormones. These factors tell me that PCOS is caused by diet and lifestyle. Carb-heavy diets and stress equal obesity and inflammation.

Obesity and inflammation equal hormonal problems. It really is that simple. What are the areas that mainstream medicine has the hardest time treating? Diet and lifestyle—there's no pill for it! So, it's no surprise that there's no mainstream cure for PCOS. This is where a keto lifestyle becomes essential to taking control of your health and fertility.

Eating keto reduces inflammation, causes your body to use up its own fat stores, while cutting sugary and carb-heavy foods that trigger insulin resistance. This is why on keto you lose weight, correct hormone imbalances, and reduce the inflammation in your reproductive organs— in both men and women—so they become capable of conception.

Though the mainstream medical world is still catching up with keto, a few recent studies have borne out what I have witnessed over the last decade of recommending keto to my patients.

A recent study comparing a low-carb diet to a low-fat diet showed that after only twelve weeks, low carb dieters lost 14% of their bodyweight and reduced their insulin levels by at least 50% while lowering their insulin resistance and triglycerides. If 14% doesn't sound like a big deal, think of it this way; if you're 200 pounds, that's a loss of 28 pounds, more than 2 pounds a week without restricting your calories. And remember, being overweight doesn't cause insulin resistance, it's the other way around. Eating sugar and carbs, not fat, makes you fat, sick, and infertile.

Another recent study looked specifically at women with PCOS who went keto for six months. Participants lost an average of 12% of their bodyweight and dropped their insulin levels by 54%. This is remarkable because the hormonal imbalances associated with PCOS make it very difficult to lose weight. Lowering body weight and decreasing insulin resistance is the key to balancing hormones so you begin to ovulate normally and become healthy enough to conceive.

Even though there's no official "cure" for PCOS, these groundbreaking studies, along with my decades of experience as a fertility doctor, affirm that a keto diet combined with healthy, stress-reducing lifestyle practices like mindful movement, meditation, and gratitude, can work together to reverse PCOS, increase your fertility, and help you grow your family.

Below I lay out simple guidelines and suggest a few effective supplements that you can use to create the right keto for PCOS plan for you:

1.Enjoy a high fat, very low carb diet.

Eating carbohydrates, especially refined carbohydrates spikes both glucose and insulin. Try setting a goal to start below 50 grams total carbohydrates per day. Spend a few days settling into your dietary routine where you're getting 70-80% of your calories from fat, then reduce your carbohydrate intake by 5-10 grams per day to increase your ketone levels while putting your fat burning capacity into overdrive.

2. Intermittent Fasting

Take advantage of the natural overnight fasting hours by skipping breakfast and eating at lunch time. When 12 hours have passed since your dinner the night before, the body officially enters a "fasted" state and will automatically begin burning fat for fuel. Benefits of intermittent fasting include fat loss, insulin sensitivity, the starvation of bad gut bacteria, neurological improvement and reduced inflammation.

3. Exercise

Mild exercising for a minimum of 30-45 minutes 4x/week will get your body burning fat and producing ketones, while cutting weight and regulating insulin.

4. Hydration

Water is critical to treating and recovering from PCOS. Water transports hormones to different parts of the body, clears harmful toxins, and carries essential nutrients to reproductive organs.

5. Natural Supplements

Though I'm skeptical of most supplements, whether plant based or synthesized, research shows that a few supplements may work together with keto to help with hormone regulation, insulin resistance, and inflammation associated with PCOS. However, since supplements are not regulated by the FDA and may interfere with other PCOS treatments, I recommend consulting with your physician before taking any of the following:

Flax seeds increase sex-hormone binding globulin levels and reduce androgen and insulin levels, making it an ideal supplement for women with PCOS.

Cinnamon comes from the bark of the cinnamon tree and has been shown to have a positive effect on insulin resistance, menstruation, and ovarian function. Intake: ½ to 1 teaspoon per day is all you need.

Apple cider vinegar (ACV) has been shown to increase insulin sensitivity in several studies, including a trial in women with PCOS. Seven women with PCOS took one tablespoon of ACV per day. After 40 days, 4 of the women resumed ovulating, 6 experienced a measurable reduction in insulin resistance, and 5 had a decrease in their LH/FSH ratio, which means they had less androgen production. Intake: 1-2 tablespoons per day.

Magnesium deficiency reduces insulin sensitivity and increases nerve excitability, leading to more stress, more tension, and more PCOS symptoms. It can be difficult to get enough magnesium on a ketogenic diet, so I recommend a general magnesium supplement.

Zinc is essential for the functioning of enzymes, hormones, and the immune system. A deficiency in zinc can cause a hormonal imbalance and make PCOS worse. Additionally, excessive or unwanted hair growth and alopecia may be improved with zinc supplements.

Inositol, a sugar alcohol compound found in foods like citrus fruits and nuts, is one of the most well-studied PCOS supplements. Most notably, inositol appears to promote ovulation and fertility. Countless studies have shown that inositol supplementation may also improve insulin resistance and decrease male hormones in the bloodstream.

Vitamin B9 is essential for women with PCOS who are trying to start a family. To improve fertility, researchers suggest that women who are at a healthy weight should take 400 micrograms of folic acid, and obese or overweight women should take 5 mg of folic acid. If a diagnosis of MTHFR gene has been determined, supplementing with L-methylfolate or 5-methyltetrahydrofolate (5-MTHF). You also can get plenty of folate by eating low-carb keto friendly leafy greens like collard greens, asparagus, kale, spinach, and cabbage.

Vitamin D is a hormone produced by the kidneys. It is vital to the endocrine system and is a very common deficiency in women with PCOS. Vitamin D and calcium may improve irregular periods and restore ovulation.

Exogenous Ketone Supplements. The term "exogenous" means anything that comes from outside the body. Therefore, all supplements are exogenous because they are ingested rather than produced by the body. The purpose of exogenous ketones is to quickly raise the level of ketone bodies circulating in your bloodstream. You can get your body into ketosis through your diet alone, but exogenous ketones are designed to speed up the process. Usually you'll find exogenous ketones in the form of powdered ketone salts. Less common are ketone esters, which are the purest form of ketones. Esters work extremely quickly, in 10 to 15 minutes as opposed to an hour for the salts, and effectively. But esters are more expensive, have a less-appealing taste, and are harder to find. The most common and accessible exogenous ketone supplement is medium-chain triglyceride (MCT) oil.

During your PCOS road to recovery, make sure to consult with a Registered Dietitian, Reproductive Endocrinologist (RE) and/or your Primary Care Physician. They can order different blood tests that will confirm how well the new diet and lifestyle are working for you.

Stephanie's Story

My name is Stephanie and my husband is Hector. We have been together for three and a half years, married for two. I have had issues with my cycles for a long time. Having PCOS and not being able to ovulate on my own, we never worried about preventing pregnancy. After getting married in July 2016, we found out that Hector was being sent overseas to Korea that October. So, we started trying right away to grow our family. Knowing it would be an issue, we started seeing Dr. Kiltz. Before my husband left the country, we stored six vials of sperm in hopes that I could keep trying for pregnancy while he was gone and knowing it could take a while. In November 2016, we were keeping an eye on a cyst I had on my ovary when we tried our first IUI. It resulted in a pregnancy that was quickly lost. I went back again for four more IUIs, all with negative results. With one vial left of sperm, and after consulting with the Dr. Kiltz, we decided to take the leap and move to IVF.

In March of 2017, after a couple weeks of stimulation, we had a lot of eggs to retrieve. Recovery from retrieval was difficult, but we ended up with seven beautiful embryos that we froze. In April, we prepared and did our first frozen transfer of two embryos. It was an exciting and scary time. We hoped and prayed that all that work and money would pay off. But the result was negative.

We tried IVF again in May and June, both times transferring two embryos. Both attempts failed. My final embryo was transferred in July 2017 and resulted in pregnancy, which I lost nine weeks later. I was left with no embryos and no baby. I consulted again with Dr. Kiltz, and since my husband wouldn't be home from Korea until that November, we took this opportunity to take a break for four months during which I finally listened to Dr. Kiltz's suggestion to try Keto. I figured what would it hurt. After being on so many medicines and supplements without success, why not give keto a shot?

In July, the week after my loss, I started keto and never looked back. I had my ratios at 75% fat, 20% protein, and 5% carbs. I was consuming less than twenty grams of carbs a day. I would say the first two weeks of switching were the most difficult. My body craved the sugar, but I never gave in.

After breaking through the cravings, I had a crazy amount of energy and mental clarity. I never felt better! The first month I was keto, I lost 30 pounds! The second month another 20. And after that 10 to 15.

In October 2017, I had laparoscopic surgery to remove the large cyst still on my ovary. I was upset because this was the third time I had to have a cyst removed due to PCOS. But after that surgery, I never had another cyst form. And even during that four-month break from fertility treatments, and while I was on keto, my cycles regulated themselves.

In November, when my husband returned, we took that month and tried on our own hoping for a miracle. Unfortunately, it didn't work, so in December, we decided to just go back to Dr. Kiltz and keep trying IUIs along with timed intercourse. At that time, my husband also decided to go Keto with me so I wouldn't be tempted by other foods. He didn't need to lose weight, but he did it just for the benefits to health and energy. He ended up losing 30 pounds and felt amazing. We continued to eat dairy because of the added protein. The instant energy and feel good boost were enough to keep us going. Add in the amazing weight loss, and how could we stop?

In December, we tried an IUI, which was unsuccessful; January and February, too. In March, we had a positive pregnancy, but unfortunately lost that too. I was so discouraged, but tried once more in April. By then, I had lost 80 pounds. That IUI was the miracle we'd been hoping for.

I'm now 35 weeks pregnant. In 2 weeks, I'll be getting induced because of some blood pressure concerns. I know for a fact that had we not stuck with Keto, we wouldn't be where we are today.

Not only did I lose 80 pounds, but my cholesterol dropped 40 points and after being on Zoloft for anxiety for fourteen years, I was able to stop taking it. I was having such great mental clarity that my doctor didn't see a need for me to be on it anymore. I also feel that the medication could have been complicating things for us. Unfortunately, I couldn't stick with Keto during pregnancy no matter how hard I tried. The high fats were hard on my stomach. I have definitely been feeling the difference not being on Keto, and I plan on starting Keto again the moment our little boy is born in a couple weeks. I'm hoping the weight I've gained during pregnancy will fall back off and Keto will also give me the energy I need for a newborn!

My advice for anyone trying Keto is NEVER give up on it; diligence is key. Also, meal prep is important and try intermittent fasting. It works and is so worth the hard work of this diet. There are also big support networks out there with advice, recipes and others going through the same process. Use these resources. You won't regret this decision, especially when the end result is a baby!

Keto for Endometriosis

Another common inflammatory disease that causes infertility is endometriosis. Like PCOS, endometriosis is correlated with hormone imbalances, in this case an excess of estrogen. Too much estrogen causes cells similar to those that make up your uterine lining (endometrium) to grow in other places in your body, including your ovaries, fallopian tubes, pelvic ligaments, and even your bowel and bladder. These cells go through the same monthly hormone induced cycles as your uterine lining, meaning they shed and bleed each time you get your period. This is why the most common symptoms of endometriosis are painful, long, and heavy periods. Sadly, cystic scarring and inflammation causes infertility in 30-40% of women with endometriosis.

Endometriosis symptoms include:

- Infertility
- Painful cramping
- Longer periods/heavy menstrual flow
- Pain during sex
- Chronic fatigue
- Nausea and/or vomiting
- Extreme hormonal aches outside of the uterus – migraines, body aches etc
- Urination and bowel problems

Like PCOS, the causes of endometriosis are still a stubborn mystery for mainstream medicine. However, new research is suggesting that endometriosis shares much in common with known autoimmune diseases, where the body begins attacking its own tissues. Hormonal imbalances and inflammation corresponding with autoimmune responses suggests that endometriosis is most likely caused by diet and lifestyle, and that at the very least, changes in diet and lifestyle are key to reversing the symptoms and giving you back your fertility.

Though mainstream medicine hasn't pinpointed the cause of endometriosis, there is a scientific consensus that exposure to toxins such as pesticides and dioxins are extreme risk factors. We know that pesticides are everywhere, and we also know that eating grass fed, local, and organic animal fats while cutting out vegetables and grains will dramatically limit exposure to pesticides, both as they occur naturally in plants as antigens and phytochemicals, and as chemicals applied to crops.

However, most people have never heard of the toxic scourge of dioxins. If you've used a tampon or pad, and if you've had coffee from a drip filter you have been exposed to dioxins. This is because dioxins are the byproduct of manufacturing bleached paper products. The EPA states that 40% to 70% of dioxins found in bleached coffee filters will be transferred into your coffee, and consequently, directly into your body! And a study by the Endometriosis Association found that 79% of rhesus monkeys exposed to dioxin developed endometriosis as a result. To limit your exposure to dioxins, I strongly recommend reusable coffee filters and unbleached menstrual products, especially products that say "dioxin free."

In addition to limiting your exposure to harmful natural and artificial pesticides, a keto way of life combats endometriosis by balancing your endocrine system. This is the system that creates hormones, including the excess estrogen that triggers endometriosis in the first place.

When you eat a carb-heavy Standard American Diet, all that sugar you're pouring into your bloodstream acts as a stressor, stimulating your adrenal glands to secrete the stress hormones cortisol and adrenaline while stimulating your pancreas to produce the hormone insulin.

As discussed earlier, the body uses insulin to turn sugar into useable energy by telling cells to accept the sugar in your bloodstream. When there's too much glucose in your bloodstream, your cells stop responding to insulin, essentially shutting the door on sugar. We call this "insulin resistance" or "pre-diabetes." When your cells stop responding to insulin, your body secretes even more insulin, bullying your cells to open their doors to let in more sugar. If you continue eating sugar, the insulin producing cells in your pancreas will burn out. Without the ability to make insulin, your body gets toxically overwhelmed by glucose, and you have diabetes—a debilitating and deadly disease.

This excess sugar that burns out your pancreas and puts you on the glucose/insulin highway to diabetes, disrupts your entire endocrine system, causing imbalances of the crucial reproductive hormones testosterone, estrogen, and progesterone that regulate ovulation. When you have endometriosis and you're not ovulating, your body stops producing progesterone. Without progesterone, your estrogen levels skyrocket, further exacerbating your endometriosis.

When you go keto, you cut out the fuel for this toxic cycle. Instead of sugar, your feeding your cells with ketones, a far superior energy source. At the same time, you're eliminating highly inflammatory plant foods like grains, legumes, and vegetables packed with phytotoxins, lectins, and plant antigens.

Caffeine, Alcohol, and your Hormones

If you have PCOS, endometriosis, or both, it's crucial that you limit your caffeine intake. A recent study of women ages 18 to 44 found that drinking coffee and other caffeinated beverages can alter levels of estrogen—but like most hormonal sensitivities the process involves complex genetic factors that we're only just discovering. For example, the study found that coffee appears to lower estrogen in white women, while in Asian women it has the reverse effect, raising estrogen levels. And because caffeine disrupts circulating androgens in both men and women, it can have dramatic effects on male fertility as well.

Alcohol is another major estrogenic toxin that can increase estrogen by 300%. The higher your level of estrogen, the more readily you absorb alcohol, but the slower you break it down, so the fatter you get. And because fat secrets estrogen, the more you drink, the harder it is to break the cycle of estrogen dominance.

A pooled analysis of data from 53 studies found for each alcoholic drink consumed per day, the relative risk of breast cancer increased by about 7 percent. Women who had 2-3 alcoholic drinks per day had a 20 percent higher risk of breast cancer compared to women who didn't drink alcohol. These outcomes are attributable to the fact that alcohol increases estrogen.

Speaking to the power of keto to break these cycles, my friend and health and wellness pioneer Maria Emmerich, shares that, "A ketogenic diet healed my addiction and anxiety around food as well as alcohol. Our cells are primarily made up of saturated fats so many people heal issues such as depression and anxiety when they begin a ketogenic lifestyle. Estrogen dominance causes low progesterone which increases anxiety and sleep issues. It is a sad snowball effect."

My keto way of life has the power to stop that snowball of depression, anxiety, and addictive carb and alcohol consumption by targeting the root of wellbeing—the health of the cells that make up every part of you and me.

Christine's Story

I had been trying to conceive for over four years. I have too many memories of going to the store to get pregnancy sticks and looking down to see the negative reading. Finally I decided to go see a fertility doctor who checked my hormone levels, and ran tests to see if my ovaries and tubes were blocked. Everything came back normal, but I just knew something was off. After consulting with other doctors, I was diagnosed with endometriosis. After speaking to numerous doctors, I met a doctor who recommended that I undergo surgery to "take a look around" to see if there was anything obvious that was causing my infertility. You can imagine my shock when he found a huge 4.5cm cyst on my left ovary that was filled with hard stuff. We did the surgery and he removed 45% of my left ovary!

That was life changing. Three months later I got pregnant and it felt like a miracle. But sadly we lost the baby. I had miscarriages on three more occasions. We didn't know why this kept happening and we were desperate. That' when we went to see Dr. Kiltz, who is literally a miracle man!

He recommended the keto diet and after following it for a couple of months I was able to maintain my current pregnancy! I believe this was because of how the diet reduces inflammation. I suffered from an the inflammatory disease called Rheumatoid arthritis my whole life. In hindsight I believe it was a causing infertility, that was until I met Dr. Kiltz who literally saved me. Without his knowledge or recommendations my baby wouldn't of survived. We're happily 34 weeks along and baby is very strong.

I believe in the Keto diet and I believe in Dr. Kiltz's practice. Love this man! I would tell other woman to talk and be open. Knowledge is power. It helped me a lot to talk about my story with other women whenever I had the chance. That's how I healed, talking and sharing and gaining knowledge. So, thank you Dr. Kiltz and your team.

B.E.B.B.I Diet: Fat is Where it's at for Fertility

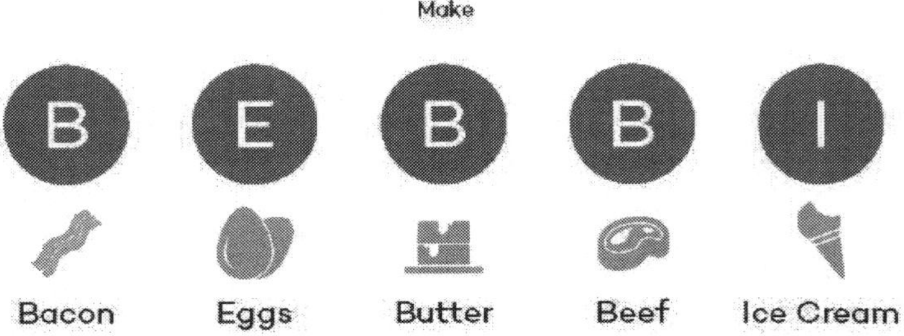
Fat is where it's at
Make
B
E
B
B
I
Bacon
Eggs
Butter
Beef
Ice Cream
the mainstays of your regular diet.

Anyone who has spoken to me has heard me repeat these five foods like a mantra; Bacon, eggs, butter, beef, and ice cream. They are the basis of Dr. Kiltz's Keto because they point to this simple truth: Our bodies require fat for energy. If we can't eat fat or make fat, we die. Unfortunately, the majority of fat we consume is industrial, man-made fat. What we really need to be eating is nature's fat—that stuff that surrounds the animal or is intertwined and marbled in every nook and cranny of the meat. Minimize the variety and simplify your meals. Eliminate pasta, bread, yogurt, milk, seeds, and nuts. Plant oils, which harden when exposed to oxygen, likely contain a multitude of plant antigens, which are harmful. Stick with high quality natural fats and use B.E.B.B.I as a rule of thumb.

Megan & Chris's Story

Shortly after getting married my husband and I decided to start a family. Two months later we were excited to find out we were pregnant and nine months later welcomed our beautiful baby girl into the world. When our daughter turned one, we decided we wanted to grow our family.

After six months of trying without any luck we decided to go to our doctor. We did some routine bloodwork and discovered that I wasn't ovulating. So we started some medications. Another ten months went by with no luck and our frustration began to grow. At this point our doctor referred us to a specialist which is when we reached out to CNY Fertility.

We quickly began working with CNY in Syracuse because the doctors and staff were so friendly. We started the process to determine the reason for our secondary infertility. It was very confusing to us considering how easy it was to conceive our first child. It was also hard because it seemed a lot of people we expressed concern to didn't understand why we were upset. A lot of the responses from people were meant to be supportive but actually hurt. Things like, "At least you have one," or "if it's not meant to be ..."

It seemed that nobody understood the pain of secondary infertility. A feeling that your choice and ability to grow your family had been taken away, especially after the joy of having our first child.

After several tests my reason for infertility was determined; I was diagnosed with premature ovarian failure. I was only 26, so this news was extremely surprising and difficult to hear. My husband and I were devastated. However, the staff and doctors were so supportive and fully explained what this meant and what our options included. After taking some time to make decisions we decided to move forward with IVF. The clinic never once tried to talk us out of our own cycle despite our condition, but after considering, we felt a donor cycle may be best.

The search then began for an egg donor and preparing my body for IVF. One of the critical steps that Dr. Kiltz strongly recommended was a keto diet. I followed keto for two months and lost 21 pounds.

Prior to the transfer we also tried acupuncture at the CNY healing arts center based on the recommendations of the staff. At this point, we were ready to begin our transfer with 4/6 donor eggs making it to transfer day. We decided to transfer 2 eggs.

Then the waiting began. The process came with so much anxiety, worry, excitement; a powerful mix of emotions. Six weeks later sitting in the waiting room as a family of three we heard the most beautiful sound; a little heartbeat.

We were now officially a family of four. The keto diet along with medications, injections, and mix of emotions continued for the next eight months. Throughout the entire process CNY was there to answer questions and provide support.

On July 26 we welcomed a beautiful baby boy into the world. We were lucky enough to have IVF work the first time and CNY made that possible. A big thank you to the CNY staff in Syracuse and to Dr. Kiltz. I really feel everything the staff did helped with our success. The acupuncture at the wonderful CNY Healing Arts Center, and the keto diet helped physically prepare my body. The positive support I received from the staff helped prepare me mentally and emotionally. Also a big thank you to the wonderful woman who donated her eggs to make my family of four possible!

Part II: The Fertile Mind

THE GRATITUDE ATTITUDE

"Cultivate the habit of being grateful for every good thing that comes to you, and to give thanks continuously. And because all things have contributed to your advancement, you should include all things in your gratitude."

— Ralph Waldo Emerson

For me, there's no better way to wake up than by greeting the day by saying, **"Thank you, God, for this awesome and amazing day you have gifted me."** If the word "God" doesn't resonate with you, that's fine, try substituting "universe." What matters is that we're acknowledging that each and every day is truly a gift. The quality of gratitude I'm expressing here comes from the deep realization that we live by the grace of our place within a vast and mysterious web of interconnections. Miraculously we are endowed with sensitive bodies, inquisitive minds, and tremendous powers of creativity with which to express our rich pallet of thoughts and emotions. Every day you wake up, you are the artist painting the masterpiece of your single, precious life. Gratitude is the feeling that arises when you realize the blessing of being you, right now, just as you are! I call this the 'gratitude attitude', and it sets me in a positive orientation to all of life as it manifests throughout my day.

Yet most of us are confused when it comes to gratitude. We think we need to achieve certain illusions of happiness, like status, wealth, power, and security before we can take a breath and appreciate all that we *are*, and not just what we have. But the truth is, happiness isn't what brings you gratitude, gratitude is what brings you happiness!

By now I hope it's clear that by happiness I'm talking about something different than an emotional state or a mood, which are temporary, in constant flux, and dependent on external events. Happiness isn't a *thing* to be acquired or a state to be achieved. Rather, true happiness comes from the *process* of how we relate to our bodies, our thoughts, and to others in each and every moment.

In this way, happiness requires a deep awareness and acceptance of the changing nature of reality. Every moment is different. Our bodies age, our thoughts and feelings ceaselessly arise and fade into new thoughts. Romances fall apart, we switch careers, friends move away, children grow up, we make new friends, find new love, and develop new interests.

If you're someone who keeps a journal, it can be a remarkable practice to turn to an entry only a few days old, let alone a few years, and notice how your concerns at this moment are completely different than the concerns that had only recently occupied your full attention, causing powerful emotions, intense thoughts, and sensations in your body.

Noticing the impermanence of your thoughts, feelings, and circumstances may at first seem a bit disenchanting. You might ask yourself, What's the point of getting so wound up and angry, so excited, and even inspired about anything if in a few days, or a few years, those same things will certainly not matter like they do now, and might not matter at all?

But it's this sense of disenchantment that can be the seed for letting go of the tired old stories that keep us bound to habits and patterns that no longer serve our highest and best good. When we see disenchantment from this perspective, it is a feeling for which we can be deeply grateful.

If I hadn't become disenchanted with the standard Western medical approach to fertility that I had devoted many years to studying and practicing, I may never have discovered the Eastern healing arts that along with Western protocols have helped countless patients conceive. Nor would I have been receptive to the power of the ketogenic diet to transform lives, and bring new life into this world.

> *"Fertility is a lifelong relationship with oneself, not a medical condition."*
>
> -Joan Borysenko, PhD

In my fertility clinics, I prescribe gratitude as an essential component of mind-body medicine—an approach based on the scientifically proven ability within each of us to re-examine our deepest held beliefs in ways that activate our powerful potential to heal ourselves.

When it comes to fertility, a change in perception from frustration and despair to gratitude has the power to effect subtle yet profound changes in your endocrine, immune, and nervous systems. As Dr. Christiane Northrup affirms, "You need to know that your ability to conceive is profoundly influenced by the complex interaction among psychosocial, psychological, and emotional factors, and that you can consciously work with this to enhance your ability to have a baby."

Gratitude practices are central to mind-body medicine because of their physical, psychological, and social benefits. The practice of gratitude has been shown to improve immune system function, regulate blood pressure, reduce stress, ameliorate aches and pains, and improve your quality of sleep. All important factors contributing to fertility in every aspect of your life.

Why Gratitude Works

Gratitude is an easy and effective way to live a **healthier, happier life.**

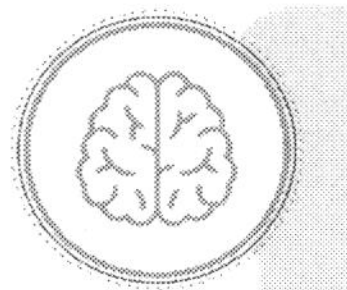

Lights up the brain's reward pathway

Floods the brain with positive chemicals, sparking brain activity critical to sleep, ograsm, mood regulation, and metabolism.

Lessens anxiety and depression symptoms

Challenging negative thought patterns calms anxiety and reduces depression.

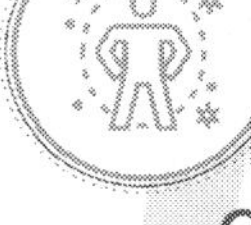

Improves physical health

Strengthens the immune system, lowers blood pressure, reduces inflammation and related symptoms like aches and pains.

Shifts the heart rhythm

Increases coherence of body functions, which facilitates higher cognitive functions, creating emotional stability and facilitating states of calm.

Gratitude is strongly and consistenly associated with GREATER HAPPINESS

Increases social connection

You can feel greater connection and feel more satisfied with friends, family, school, community and yourself.

Increases heart rate variability

Heart patients who practice gratitude show better moods, better sleep, less fatigue and lower levels of inflammatory biomarkers related to cardiac health.

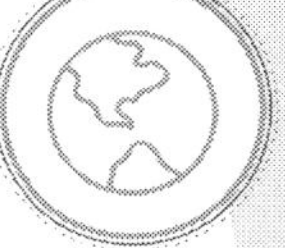

Increases empathy & compassion

The more gratitude we generate within ourselves the more likley we are to act pro-socially toward others, which in turn causes others to feel grateful, setting off a cascade of positivity

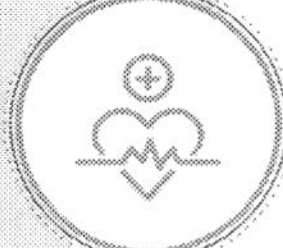

Increases resilience

Helps you bounce back from stressful events and helps you deal with adversity by acting as a buffer against internalizing symptoms.

The #1 Way to practice gratitude is by writing in a **Gratitude Journal.**

"The thoughts manifest as the word; The words manifest as the deed; The deeds develop into habits, And habit hardens into character."

-Buddha

Accepting and being grateful for the fact that reality is always changing helps us to let go of patterns that put a strangle hold on our innate freedom and creativity. If everything is always changing, then it's foolish to hold on to anything too tightly, including our current beliefs and habits. It can be helpful to reflect on how we humans are hard-wired for habits. And almost all of us have some habit we are struggling to change. We don't have to get down on ourselves, nor do we have to identify with our habits. But it is important to acknowledge that we become addicted to and identify with all forms of familiarity, not only to familiar pleasures, but to familiar ways of suffering.

Beginning with the food we eat and extending here to the practice of gratitude, my *keto way of life* is the blueprint for changing our habits i.e., our relationships, to every aspect of our lives. To be clear, I'm not suggesting that we push away our thoughts and feelings. After all, our ability to think and feel, to become inspired, angry, sad, to fall in love, and strive for our goals are all perfect expressions of who we are in this and every moment. I'm suggesting that we can be grateful for these parts of ourselves without identifying with them.

This shift from "identifying with" your thoughts and feelings to "noticing and being with" your thoughts and feelings entails a subtle shift in perspective and a physiological change in your brain. It's natural if you're having trouble completely getting it right now. It's an experience that you can't think your way into. Rather, it evolves from our practice.

You will develop an experiential sense of what I'm talking about once you begin the practices I introduce later in this chapter. In the meantime, a little more explanation might be helpful: You can feel sadness, and even say "I am sad," without meaning "I am a sad person." And you can make the language you use around difficult emotions a powerful part of your gratitude and mindfulness routines. Rather than saying "I am sad," try saying, "There is sadness in me." The same goes for positive emotions. When we say, "There is joy in me," we don't beat ourselves up when we're feeling like we've *lost* our joy in the face of some new challenge life throws our way.

By changing how we talk about ourselves we're acknowledging that being human means being available to the full spectrum of experience, the highs and the lows, without getting too bent out of shape or attached to any passing feeling. From this realization comes a deep and abiding sense of peace and acceptance, which is the true root of true happiness.

The key to understanding this shift is to recognize that it's not the feelings themselves that cause us suffering, but our attachments and resistances to our feelings. Realizing that attachment is the root of suffering allows us to be more grateful for all of our emotions, thoughts, and physical sensations.

In the poem *The Guest House,* the 13th century mystic poet, Rumi, beautifully conveys how grateful acceptance of our feelings in the awareness of change can make us available to the innate wisdom hidden in each and every one of us.

This being human is a guest house.
Every morning a new arrival.

A joy, a depression, a meanness,
some momentary awareness comes
As an unexpected visitor.

Welcome and entertain them all!
Even if they're a crowd of sorrows,
who violently sweep your house
empty of its furniture,
still treat each guest honorably.
He may be clearing you out
for some new delight.

The dark thought, the shame, the malice,
meet them at the door laughing,
and invite them in.

Be grateful for whoever comes,
because each has been sent
as a guide from beyond.

-Rumi

"Piglet noticed that even though he had a very small heart, it could hold a rather large amount of gratitude."

—A.A. Milne, Winnie-the-Pooh

I know we're covering a lot of ground here. Gratitude is an extremely rich part of being a human that is deeply embedded in the connections between our minds, bodies, and emotions. In other words, *when we practice gratitude, we become gratitude.* I call this experience the *Mind Body Smile.* It is my hope that as you try the gratitude practices I introduce later in this chapter and integrate them with the other parts of my keto way of life, you will find your way back to these words and feel them ringing clear and true in every cell of your being.

Cultivating gratitude supports and sets the tone for every part of our lives. And the beautiful thing about gratitude is that it is available to all of us. Its presence is felt and expressed by all people, of all cultures, across the world, and throughout time.

We are all hard-wired for deep and abiding gratitude. But we won't activate this inherent gratitude attitude and all its benefits, nor share them with everyone in our lives, unless we nurture the seeds of gratitude through practice. Though the effects of practicing gratitude can be immediate, they don't appear magically, and they get stronger over time. Once activated and set, the gratitude attitude gains momentum and will continue to enhance your fertility along with your general physical and psychological well-being for years.

When it comes to bringing new life into this world, it's hard to think of a more powerful and valuable way of being to pass on to our future generations. By beginning your gratitude practices right now, you can create a ripple effect of well-being that spreads from you into the world at large. Just as normal smiles are contagious, the *Mind Body Smile* that comes from gratitude is absolutely irresistible.

GRATITUDE PRACTICES

> *"When I started counting my blessings, my whole life turned around."*
>
> —*Willie Nelson*

Gratitude journaling is the gold standard of gratitude practices. It's been used in hundreds of studies worldwide bearing out gratitude's myriad benefits. Its positive effects on our brains, bodies, attitudes, and relationships are incontrovertible. The beauty of gratitude journaling is in its simplicity. All you need is a journal and something to write with, or a dedicated word processing file on your computer.

You can begin quite simply by writing down three things that you are grateful for in your life three days a week. The three-day approach protects us from the sense of pressure many of us feel towards adding daily routines and the shame we feel if we forget or aren't able to see them through. I get it. Our lives are super busy, and the practice of gratitude is here to help us feel less stress and more positive about life. Running six fertility clinics across two states and two countries, some days I only have time for my morning affirmation: "Thank you, God, for this awesome and amazing day you have gifted me." It's no substitute, but it's a great tool to keep the fire of gratitude lit.

So, start with three days a week. As you begin to feel the momentum of the gratitude attitude building, naturally increase the frequency of your journaling by a day or two. If you find yourself journaling every day while still finding more things to be grateful for each day, bravo! If not, that's totally fine too. There's no one size fits all. And just as there's no right or wrong frequency for gratitude journaling, no one can tell you what you should or shouldn't be grateful for. The things we feel grateful for are unique to each and every one of us, and they change from day to day, just as we do. This brings us to another benefit of gratitude journaling. For many people, it doubles as a daily diary that you can look back on in order to gain deeper insights into the themes and patterns appearing in your lives, all through the nurturing and inspiring lens of the gratitude attitude.

When just starting out, it can be helpful to have a few prompts, so here's a short list taken from some of my own gratitude reflections:

- What is there about a challenge you are experiencing right now that you can be thankful for?
- Who has done something to help you this week for which you are grateful? How can you thank them?
- What was the last great experience you had in nature?
- What was the most delicious ketogenic meal you've had this last week?
- How is your life today different than it was one year ago, and what about these changes are you grateful for?
- List three people in your life you find it difficult to get along with and write down a positive quality you see in each of them that you are grateful for.
- What is something new you've learned this week that you are grateful for?
- What music did you listen to this week that you are grateful to have heard?
- Something that made you smile today?
- Something funny that made you laugh?
- A favorite place you've visited?
- A modern invention that you rely on and are grateful for?

It's ok if you don't have answers to any these questions, they're just here to help get the juices flowing.

GUIDED GRATITUDE MEDITATION

Guided gratitude meditations are another proven way to activate the power of gratitude.

Daily practice

Consistency is key to unlocking the power of any meditation just as with each of the practices that are part of my keto way of life, including of course, the keto diet. When people ask how much meditation they need to truly feel its effects, I liken it to the activities we use to keep our body healthy. Your body responds optimally to a few hours of intentional activity each week. The same goes for your mind. To explore and enjoy the full benefits of guided meditation, it's best to commit to a daily or twice daily practice of at least 20 minutes at a time. The 20-minute suggestion is based on the fact that our brains take on average 15 minutes to fully focus on any one task. Meditators, especially when just starting out, often remark that they didn't really feel like they were truly meditating until the last 5 minutes of their practice. But in truth, you are meditating from the moment you begin the practice. Simply noticing without judgment the way the mind latches on to thoughts and distractions is a powerful way to expand your awareness, and it is the principle of mindfulness meditation.

Same time, same place

As I discussed earlier, we are creatures of habit, and when it comes to practicing meditation, we can use this to our advantage. By choosing the same time and place to meditate each day, we are priming our bodies and brains to drop into meditative focus more quickly and deeply. I recommend finding a place in your home where you intuitively feel comfortable. It's best if it's somewhere private, insulated from physical distractions, bright lights, and sound. That said, it's important to give ourselves and our loved ones a break. Our lives are busy. Many of us have rambunctious families with members who aren't familiar with meditation, and they may have difficulty understanding the boundaries we need to establish. Most of us don't have the luxury of escaping to a cave—real or metaphorical. So, for me, I find it liberating to make the distractions themselves a part of the practice. When a distraction occurs, I view it as an opportunity to strengthen my practice by gently and lovingly turning my attention back to the object of meditative focus as I say to the distraction, "Thank you precious teacher." As we deepen our practices, we will discover that the true hallmark of effective meditation is that we can bring it with us into any situation. Any situation, no matter how challenging, is truly our precious teacher. Though it's helpful to have an undistracted meditative environment especially when we're starting out, there is nothing precious about the environment itself. As with the rest of reality, it's healthy to not grasp on to it too tightly.

Posture

Often meditation teachers make a big deal about sitting in a pretzel (i.e., lotus position). This can feel like a roadblock for beginners, but if we go back to the earliest meditation manuals, we find that there was nothing particularly spiritual about sitting this way. The lotus posture was simply a common way of sitting among yogis that was most comfortable and stable for long periods of time. The most important element of your meditation posture is that it be comfortable. Though I have found the traditional posture where you sit cross-legged with a straight back and neck on a Japanese meditation pillow called a *zafu*—this raises your butt, taking pressure off your hips and knees and keeping your back straighter—to be most comfortable for me, I've meditated while sitting in chairs, lying down, on the couch, in the car—and they all work just fine. However, the straighter your back, the better, since this helps open up your breathing. Other than that, find what works best for you.

Zero judgment

There is no right or wrong way to meditate. There are no grades, no external judges, and nothing to judge. Are you showing up and giving it your best effort? That's all that matters. When we first start out, it can feel like we're just riding the rollercoaster of our distracted minds but for only brief moments when we step off into more focused states of awareness. On the deepest level, that's all meditation ever is—in the contrast between riding our thoughts and being aware of them, we are becoming directly aware of the nature of our own minds.

The more often you practice, the less time you spend on the rollercoaster. But for nearly everyone except perhaps the greatest masters, the rollercoaster never fully stops. Guided gratitude meditation adds a specific flavor to meditation by taking us on a journey into the depths of one very powerful quality of being. But the meditative principle remains the same: while practicing, you are exploring what it is to be you through sustained, intentional, focus. If we get frustrated by distraction, simply notice the frustration, then *gently* and l*ovingly* shift your awareness back to the object of focus. For many people, it is helpful to recite the words "gently and lovingly return my awareness back to the moment of gratitude." This process of relating gently to frustration is how we let it go. There's a profound difference between resisting and grasping and letting go. As you meditate, see if you can detect this difference. Strengthening your ability to let go and return to your calm, focused awareness while in meditation directly translates to your ability to do so in each and every life situation.

GUIDED GRATITUDE PRACTICE

1.Settle into in a relaxed posture. Keeping your eyes open but allowing your gaze to soften and rest, feel the pressure of your body against the ground. Inhale for 5 seconds, hold for 5 seconds, release your breath slowly for 10 seconds. Repeat this sequence of breathing 3 times.

Think about something in your life you are very grateful for. Notice where you can feel that in your body. Inhale for 5 seconds, hold for 5 seconds, release your breath slowly for 10 seconds.

Notice any sensations in your immediate surroundings. What do you smell, taste, touch, see, hear? **Say to yourself: "For this, I am grateful."** Inhale for 5 seconds, hold for 5 seconds, release your breath slowly for 10 seconds.

Next, call forth into your mind an image of someone who you effortlessly feel love for—a close friend, a family member, your partner. **Say to yourself, "For this, I am grateful."** Inhale for 5 seconds, hold for 5 seconds, release your breath slowly for 10 seconds.

Next, turn your attention onto yourself: You are a unique and exquisite being. You are able to feel a rich spectrum of emotions; you can communicate with others,\; you have a splendid imagination that allows you to learn from the past and prepare for the future; and you have the resolve to focus right here and now on the gift of being you at this very moment. **Say to yourself: "For this, I am grateful."** Inhale for 5 seconds, hold for 5 seconds, release your breath slowly for 10 seconds.

Finally, rest in the realization that your life is a precious gift from the universe. You are resilient in the face of challenge and gracious in the face of success. **Say to yourself: "For this, I am grateful."** Inhale for 5 seconds, hold for 5 seconds, release your breath slowly for 10 seconds.

Heather & Roy's Story

Before my husband and I got married we knew we wanted children more than anything else in life. What we didn't know was how hard that was going to be. We tried on our own for eight months. And month after month we watched each test come up negative. We finally decided to seek help. We met with a fertility specialist where we were living and he wanted us to do timed intercourse with Clomid. Our doctor assured us we would have no issues and we would be celebrating very soon. We followed the instructions but months went by with no cause for celebration. My husband and I really started to feel the pressure and stress of not conceiving.

We ended up moving to another state and seeking a new doctor who sent me for all kinds of tests and bloodwork. That's when we discovered that I had PCOS and a very large cyst on my right ovary. This lead to surgery to remove the cyst. Once I healed we were back to trying for our miracle. This doctor wanted us to try three cycles with Femera, along with timed intercourse. Three months later we still had no reason to celebrate. The doctor decided an IUI would be our next approach. We ended up doing seven IUI cycles, each yielding a negative result. We were devastated.

The doctor told us that at this point our only option was IVF. My husband and I talked about it and met with the medical team to figure things out. That meeting didn't go very well. For one treatment we were looking at a cost of around $20,000. Having a baby seemed so far out of reach for us. We went home upset and I started to search around for other options. That's when I found CNY fertility.

I scheduled a consult with Dr. Kiltz, and our conversation was great. He strongly recommended that I try Keto diet prior to IVF. We were skeptical but obviously very motivated, and after only a couple months both my husband and I each lost over 30 lbs. Feeling healthy and energized we were ready to begin our treatment. I had all kinds of bloodwork done once and I began taking oral and injection medications. In October of 2017 we traveled six hours to the CNY Fertility center in Syracuse Ny for my retrieval. We ended up with twelve embryos. However, I had overstimulated, and was unable to transfer any at that time. I spent the next few weeks healing and trying to get better. In November we were ready for our transfer.

I took my transfer meds and then we traveled back to CNY. This was the day that all our preparation with keto and all the procedures lead up to! The doctors transferred two AA embryos into me. Six days after the transfer we got our first positive! After four frustrating years of trying and seeing negative after negative this first positive was surreal. We were overwhelmed with joy. Thanks to CNY for helping us start our family. We couldn't be more thankful.

Fertile Failure

FERTILIZE THE UNIVERSE, MAKE SOME MISTAKES!

"I have not failed. I've just found 10,000 ways that won't work."
– Thomas A. Edison

Don't let fear of failure hold you back. If you're not making mistakes, you're not trying anything new. If you're not trying anything new, you're not growing. I like to say that mistakes are fertilizer. Fertilizer is good for the soil of all life—yours, your children's, and the lives of everyone who knows you, and even those who you may never meet, yet who are part of the vast ecology of human consciousness. Fertilizer gives renewed creative power and strength to the seedlings that grow out of it. Failure is fertilizer for life. Failing makes us stronger, smarter, more motivated, and hones our focus. The next time you feel defeated by circumstance or you make a mistake, suffer folly or foible—and trust me you will—instead of saying, "I failed," try saying "I fertilized." There's a lot more truth to the latter!

When I first took up painting, my daughter told me I wasn't very good (and frankly, she was right), but that didn't stop me from trying. I worked hard at it, and over time saw I great improvement, and most importantly, I found great joy in the act of painting itself, independent of whether or not any single painting met my own highest standards or the personal preferences of others. And herein lies one of the keys to having a fertile mindset when it comes to failure:

the experience of failure, and conversely, of success are completely dependent on how you see things.

As long as I can remember, I've enjoyed an innate curiosity towards the power of our beliefs (both conscious and unconscious) to shape our experience and change our lives in both emotional and material ways. As an artist, doctor, entrepreneur, and practitioner of conscious living, I've become deeply inspired by the power we have to change our beliefs. I've experienced this first-hand in my own life and witnessed it work for countless patients.

If I look back far enough, I can see that my interest in the power of belief comes from growing up with some significant hardships. As I detailed earlier in these pages, my parents, though deeply loving and supportive, suffered failed businesses, lost houses, and at one point my father was in jail. I myself was dyslexic, I was in a gang, got into trouble, failed classes. Even as I became an adult, got into med school, became a doctor, I encountered my fair share of challenges—missed out on residencies I thought I wanted; didn't get positions I thought were important to my career; business and romantic partnerships fell apart; and I became disenchanted with aspects of western medicine.

But instead of taking each of these failures as a sign that I wasn't good enough or smart enough or that something was inherently wrong with me, I viewed them as profound learning experiences. I asked, *what can I take away from this challenge that will help me grow as a person, while at the same time showing me how to overcome similar challenges in the future?*

Not surprisingly, the answers to both the personal and circumstantial questions were deeply intertwined. What I discovered is that from our deepest and most personal realms of artistic expression and spirituality, to our close relationships and family, to the collective realms of work and community, our reality is a direct manifestation of the beliefs we hold about ourselves and the world around us.

Perhaps the most fundamental beliefs we carry about ourselves, the ones that cut to the core of who we are and make the difference between *growing* rather than *stagnating* in the face of our fears, have to do with how we respond to failure.

No one has done more work towards understanding the fruits that grow from the fertilizer of failure than Stanford psychologist Carol Dweck. Her real-world research over the last two decades looking at the power of mindsets for individuals, relationships, and businesses has revealed that the most important factor for success is not "innate" talent or intelligence, but rather attitude and mindset.

In the previous chapter on gratitude, I talked about how a *gratitude attitude* has the power to transform every life experience into a flow of moments erupting with grace and insight. Now I want to share how we can deepen this teaching about attitude, especially when it comes to facing seeming failure. And I know that infertility can feel like the biggest failure of all.

Let's begin by examining what Carol Dweck identified as our two basic mindsets, which she refers to as the "fixed mindset" and the "growth mindset." If we have a "fixed mindset," we assume that our character, intelligence, and creative abilities are static givens that can't be changed. With a fixed mindset, success is the affirmation of your inherent intelligence. Striving for success and avoiding failure at all costs becomes a way of grasping onto your sense of being smart or skilled. On the other hand, a "growth mindset" thrives on challenge and views failure not as evidence of a lack of intelligence, but as a powerful catalyst for growth and for increasing our abilities in every area of our lives each and every day.

Two Mindsets

Carol S. Dweck, Ph.D.

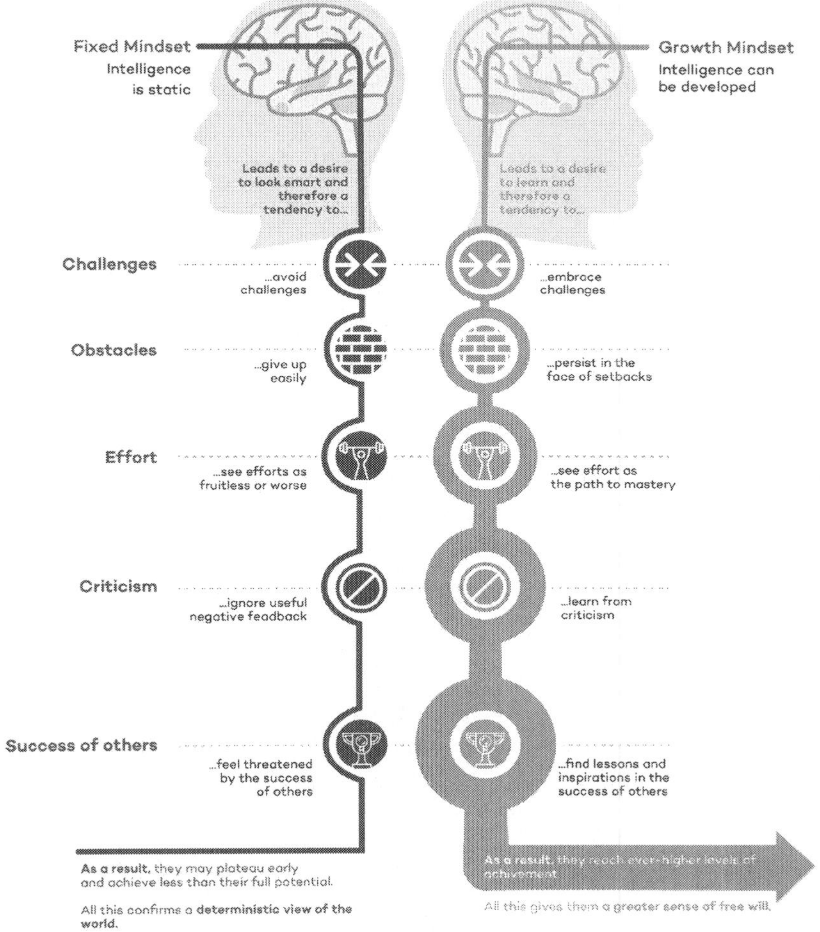
Fixed Mindset
Intelligence is static
Growth Mindset
Intelligence can be developed
Leads to a desire to look smart and therefore a tendency to...
Leads to a desire to learn and therefore a tendency to...
Challenges
...avoid challenges
...embrace challenges
Obstacles
...give up easily
...persist in the face of setbacks
Effort
...see efforts as fruitless or worse
...see effort as the path to mastery
Criticism
...ignore useful negative feedback
...learn from criticism
Success of others
...feel threatened by the success of others
...find lessons and inspirations in the success of others
As a result, they may plateau early and achieve less than their full potential.
All this confirms a deterministic view of the world.
As a result, they reach ever-higher levels of achivement.
All this gives them a greater sense of free will.

REALITY > FICTION

As a culture, we Americans all too often base our self-worth on the illusion of innate intelligence measured by IQ and affirmed by stellar grades in fancy schools. And we beat ourselves up for not achieving all these things and comparing ourselves to others who have what we don't. We neurotically measure our "success" in life in terms of accumulated financial wealth. I find it liberating to blast holes in these false narratives with a few quick shots of realty. For one, the IQ test was created by French psychologist Alfred Binet, not to measure intelligence, but to identify how and for whom the French school system was failing. Not only does IQ measure only a very narrow spectrum of cognitive ability, poverty lowers IQ by an average of 13 points, which can be the difference between someone scoring as average or impaired, or the difference between scoring as merely average and regional genius.

Number two, the single most powerful factor for success in life is not intelligence or even academic achievement—it's having the dumb luck of being born to wealthy parents. As a matter of fact, people who come from wealthy families and don't even go to college are *twice* as likely to achieve high levels of socio-economic status (SES) than people who come from humble means and *earn* a college degree. Among affluent families, a kindergartner with test scores in the bottom half has a 7 in 10 chance of reaching high SES among his or her peers as a young adult, while a disadvantaged kindergartner with top-half test scores only has a 3 in 10 chance. Add to this the fact that doggedness and grit are better predictors of success than IQ, and we have to re-write the entire story of success in America. I point to my own story of coming from a humble beginnings as an example of what you can achieve from a mixture of luck and hard work. So if you're struggling with fertility, stay with the program. My keto way of life is here because I've seen it work for countless patients. The first few days may be tough, but you will get the hang of it, and you will take control of your fertility.

DO. OR DO NOT. THERE IS NO TRY

Speaking of grit, when I'm faced with what feel like insurmountable challenges, I often think of Master Yoda's famous words, "Do. Or do not. There is no try." These are the last words of wisdom the Jedi Master gives Luke before he attempts to raise his X-wing fighter from the swamp. This lightning bolt of wisdom entered Luke and showed him the power of being completely focused on the present moment. I see the X-wing fighter not as an object but as a metaphor for the self. With total presence, focus, and determination, you can lift yourself from the swamp of delusions and false beliefs.

I poke holes in the common narratives of success and self-worth not to discourage you from seeking financial stability or the empowerments and personal pleasures of education. On the contrary, I consider myself to be a passionate lifelong learner, an attitude that's responsible for nearly everything I'd label as truly successful in my life, from the deep caring connections I enjoy with family, friends, patients, and colleagues, to the growth of my fertility practice, to all the tools for wellbeing and fertility that I'm sharing with you in this book.

ONLY CONNECT!

> *"Only connect! That was the whole of her sermon. Only connect the prose and the passion, and both will be exalted, and human love will be seen at its height. Live in fragments no longer."*
>
> -E.M. Forster

I want to pause here for a moment to emphasize why throughout this book I talk a lot about cultivating, deepening, and improving our connections and relationships, both to ourselves and to others. It's no stretch to say that the purpose of life is to continually deepen these relationships, and that we can determine the value of anything we do based on whether it supports or impairs our process of deepening our connection to ourselves and to others. I believe connection is so important because on the most basic evolutionary level, humans are social creatures. From the moment we're born, if we don't connect with other humans we die. And our dependence on connection isn't just limited to infancy. For the vast majority of human history, to be ostracized from the tribe or village was to be handed a death sentence.

In the modern world, if we're isolated, we have infrastructure in place to keep most of us from dying of starvation and exposure. Yet feelings of loneliness and despair are at historic levels. In 2018, Health insurer Cigna surveyed 20,000 adults and found that 54% of them said they feel like no one actually knows them well. 56% of respondents said the people they surround themselves with "are not necessarily with them," and 40% said they "lack companionship," that their "relationships aren't meaningful," and that they feel "isolated from others."

This epidemic of loneliness during a time when we're supposedly more connected than ever, calls into question what we're connecting to? Why? And what's it doing to our minds and bodies? Our need to cultivate deep, meaningful, and loving connections is important to consider when preparing to have children of your own.

JUNK FOOD FOR OUR SOULS

By now, most of us know how advertising is aimed at making us feel inadequate so we buy the thing that's supposed to make us feel better. But there's a new kind of advertising that's even more insidious than standard commercials and print ads. The most valuable commodity in this age of information is your attention.

Attention is valuable because the longer you spend on any online media, be it a news website or social media platforms like Facebook and twitter, the more advertisements they can send your way. This is how these websites make money. You don't pay them for their content, but they get paid by other businesses to 'serve' you advertisements. These platforms are smart, and what they've learned from all the data they've collected about our media consuming habits is that our attention is most riveted to stories and content that scares us and makes us angry. They are praying on our most basic survival instincts, sowing mistrust, stress, and division just to so they can feed you one more advertisement for a product or service you don't need.

Yet we live in a world that has never been more cooperative, less violent, and filled with material abundance. As cognitive psychologist, Steven Pinker points out in his book *Enlightenment Now,* for the first time in human history, humans are more likely to die of suicide than of violence. But you'd never imagine this to be the case when looking at your FB news feed.

All too often our response to the constant stream of attention-capturing darkness, loneliness, self-loathing, and mistrust is to sooth ourselves with sugar in the form of processed foods I call "carbo-caine."

The practices in this book from diet, to mindset, to meditation are meant to be a medicine that helps us reconnect with ourselves. The more attuned we become to our own minds and bodies, the more deeply, joyfully, and meaningfully we can connect with others. And the more love we can bring into the world as we grow our families. In many ways, my keto way of life is my *connection* way of life.

FOCUS ON WHAT'S IN YOUR CONTROL

My purpose in exposing both fixed ideas of intrinsic self-worth and external ideas of success as flimsy and mostly out of our hands, is to encourage you to become aware of the parts of yourself that are truly within your control. Though we can't choose what happens to us in this lifetime, we can choose how we respond to whatever is happening in each moment.

One of the most valuable things we can choose is to cultivate a **growth mindset** that rewards us with a passion for learning rather than a painful yearning for approval. A growth mindset allows us to see failures, foibles, and follies in all their glory—as opportunities to reach our highest potential!

Unfortunately, we don't all get to have a Master Yoda by our side, guiding us with encouragement, centuries of wisdom, and the protection of the mysterious "force." Yet, an extensive body of research, along with six decades of being me, and more than twenty-years of helping people achieve the goal of growing their families, makes clear that within each and every one of us there exists a bridge between a fixed mindset and a growth mindset. This bridge, should we choose to cross it, is built from our own self-awareness.

SELF-AWARENESS IS THE BRIDGE TO GROWTH

> *"Our outer world will always be a reflection of our inner world. Our level of success is always going to parallel our level of personal development. Until we develop time each day to developing ourselves into the person we need to be to create the life we want, success is always going to be a struggle to attain."*
>
> -Hal Elrod

Becoming self-aware means we know what motivates us to take actions and make decisions. It means we recognize our emotional reactions to every circumstance either positive or negative. We notice the sensations these circumstances bring about in our bodies, how they connect with our emotions, how our emotions manifest as beliefs about ourselves and others, and how these beliefs shape our thoughts and actions. *Through self-awareness, we come to recognize what it is to be ourselves in any given moment.*

You cannot change who you are without self-awareness. We cannot change what we cannot see. Without self-awareness, there's no way to understand how to address our own strengths and weaknesses. The purpose of changing our mindset is to discover where and how we can take steps to grow. And this process becomes especially important as we take steps to grow our families.

KETO AS A FOUNDATION OF AWARENESS

Enjoying a ketogenic diet is a powerful foundation for self-awareness. Keto helps us become sensitive to how food affects us on both physical and emotional levels. It reveals to us how we frequently use food to manage our emotions, just like a drug, and mostly in unhealthy ways.

I bet you've heard the saying, "eating your feelings." "Feelings" here almost always refers to sadness, loneliness, and frustration. And "eating" usually means consuming loads of sugary, processed, junk food. This is because when we eat sugar, we're stimulating the same parts of our brains that light-up when we spend time with family and close friends.

KICKING THE CARBO-CAINE

This is one of the reasons why sugar is so addictive. When I encourage friends and patients to base their diet on bacon, eggs, butter, beef, and keto ice cream while removing carbohydrates and sugar, most worry they won't be able to do it. Carbs and sugar have a deep emotional grip on many of us. You're not imagining it. I refer to carbs as "carbo-caine".

Like cocaine, carbs are addictive. Eating carbs affects the pleasure centers in the brain just like a drug. High carb consumption spikes insulin which allows tryptophan to enter the brain and make serotonin, the feel-good neurotransmitter. Eating carbs quite literally makes us happy, but only temporarily, and then we crash! A steady diet of high carbs and sugar will create a host of problems that affect your daily enjoyment of life and can shorten your lifespan while dramatically impairing your fertility.

By contrast, when we're eating a keto diet based on healthy fats combined with intermittent feasting, we kick our sugar addictions and create a potent space for awareness of every other part of life—our friends, family, hobbies, careers etc.—when previously our awareness was constricted to the act of chasing the next carb-fix.

For most people who practice my keto way of life, the emotional insights and stabilization that takes place are far more profound than the changes to their physique. My keto way of life brings into focus the entire picture of who you are, not just what you look like.

Ramona & Stepan's Story

I am 34 years old and I started fertility treatments when I was 28. When we first looked for help, we went to a clinic where we did 4 rounds of Clomid with a trigger shot, then two IUI's, but none of it worked.

After that, we decided to take a break for two years. When I was ready to try again, we came to CNY Fertility. My husband and I were both tested, and it turned out I was the one having trouble getting pregnant. We started with IUI right away, and the first few attempts came back negative. When our final attempt was positive, it was the happiest day of my life. We went for an ultrasound and discovered I was carrying twins.

Soon after I was shocked to find out that one of the twins didn't make it. But the second twin was strong, and nine months later we had our son Zayn. It's was the best moment of our lives. We talked and decided we were going to try on our own to get pregnant. After one year of trying, we ended up getting pregnant but had a miscarriage right away. We were devastated. So, we talked and decided we were going to go back to CNY Fertility to undergo two more attempts—if it worked, good. If not, we will just be grateful for our first son. Both attempts came back negative.

While I was at the clinic, Dr. Kiltz talked about the KETO diet and encouraged me to try it, telling me with confidence that it would work. I didn't believe it, but I had nothing to lose so I gave it a try. At that time, I was 5'8" and weighed 265 lbs. After doing KETO for 6 months, I went down to 177lbs. That's a loss of 88 lbs, all from eating mostly fat! I was feeling physically great and emotionally happy. But then one night I felt weird, so I called my husband and told him to buy me pregnancy test. In the morning the test read positive! We were in shock. We told each other we were going to pretend like I wasn't pregnant because we were so scared something bad would happen. Thankfully, nine months later I gave birth to my second son, Iden, my second miracle. I am so happy and so blessed and thankful to CNY Fertility and all doctors and nurses there. Without any of you and without keto, we would not have these two beautiful boys.

The Craving Mind vs. The Caring Mind

"And now that you don't have to be perfect, you can be good."
–John Steinbeck

Practicing a ketogenic diet works hand-in-hand with the other self-awareness practices in this book to give us more control and choice over our addictive and unhealthy habits. To the extent that *we are our habits,* this newly forged power of choice allows us to fundamentally change who we are, making it possible for our truest, freest, most present and empowered versions of ourselves to emerge.

As I alluded to earlier in this chapter, as you grow in self-awareness, you begin to notice how your experience of being you is formed in large part by the ways you habitually react to the events and circumstances life throws your way. For most of us, our default way of going through life is to unconsciously, emotionally react. We then act according to our emotional reactions and identify with our reactions and actions.

Finally, to protect our sense of self-identity, we begin justifying and defending our reactions and actions. Through all this, we dull our self-reflective instincts with external distractions, by ingesting substances like junk food, alcohol, and narcotics, and letting our minds wander in fantasies of the future or ruminations on the past.

In this chain of actions and reactions, there is no space for awareness, no reflection, and therefore no choice. Without self-awareness, we're sleepwalking through life. We are being dreamed, rather than being the dreamers of our own lives. And as you're preparing to bring new life into the world, it's the perfect opportunity to wake up to your own life.

The first stage in waking up is to ask how this dream we're stuck in has come to be? To answer this, we have to start at the very beginning. From the time you were born, and recent studies suggest that this happens even in utero, you absorbed models of how to react to reality from the people closest to you. For most of us this means our parents.

These early childhood experiences are more than just memories, they are models of behavior that we refer back to and repeat so often that they come to form our character and personality. Our minds and bodies instinctually download these behavior models similar to how computers download software. As with computer software, these models act as instructions that help us interpret, identify, and respond to the flow of information (physical and emotional phenomenon that is constantly bombarding our senses). "Say please and thank you," and "Look both ways before crossing the street," are common primary models, just as "Self-awareness is the bridge to a growth mindset," is a model, albeit one that many of you may have only just come across.

We also come into the world with a set of hardware upon which the software of consciousness runs. This hardware is our genetic inheritance, i.e., our DNA. It's still up for debate as to how much influence genes and models of behavior have over one another. But as a fertility doctor working closely with thousands of emotionally charged bodies and minds, it's been my first-hand experience that increasing our self-awareness and consequently changing our beliefs, intentions, and habits unleashes tremendous power to heal and transform our entire self— mind, body, and soul, while making fertility a reality for people who never thought it possible.

A NEW PICTURE OF YOU

My hope is that by reading this book, a new picture of you is beginning to develop. A picture in which you begin to see yourself as you truly are: a dynamic bundle of interactions between numerous and changing experiences taking place within and around you. In Buddhist terminology, this picture of what it is to be a person is called *dependent origination.* Dependent origination describes how your physical sensations, emotions, thoughts, and memories are all working in concert to create the experience of being an "I".

When we view ourselves from the perspective of dependent origination, we can see how having a growth mindset as opposed to a fixed mindset isn't merely just a helpful mental model for turning life's lemons into lemonade. It's a way to truly live in accord with what you are on the deepest level. Nothing about who you think you are is fixed. Every part of you is growing and changing. This is includes your fertility.

Of course, some parts of us are much harder to consciously change than others. And by change, I don't mean we become completely different people overnight. Rather, the changes we experience when practicing my keto way of life result from accumulated shifts of habit, perspective, and belief that produce more positive emotions and pleasurable physical states, while forming a foundation for choices and actions that bring about deep caring connections to ourselves, others, and the world at large.

Yet, because of the prevailing models of success, failure, and self-worth that we're force-fed by society, media, parents, and peers, it's all too easy to lose sight of the power we have to manifest our most creative, joyful, and loving potential.

What's more, we humans are hardwired with a tendency to perpetuate our experiences of limitation and suffering, a tendency that's encoded in the very structure of our minds. As Anil K. Seth, the world's preeminent researcher of consciousness points out, the twin goals of consciousness are to conserve energy while maintaining homeostasis. Simply put, this means our minds are constantly comparing our present experiences to memories of similar things we've experienced in the past, while using memories to interpret what we're experiencing.

Seeing the present through the past and acting accordingly is why so many of us get stuck in cycles of familiar experiences, even if they're unpleasant, limiting, and destructive. We are creatures of habit, for better and for worse. On the flip side, we are also extremely adaptable. How we adapt and change is mainly a matter of finding and being open to new models of being.

I believe the ketogenic diet is the foundation for being able to adapt and change in the deepest ways possible. We know that when we eat mostly fat, the resulting ketones are a more sustainable, efficient, and energy rich fuel than carbohydrates. More energy equals more consciousness. Keto is quite literally consciousness expanding.

At the same time, a keto diet relieves us of our most persistent and harmful cravings. From the perspective of dependent origination, release from cravings means a fundamental shift in who we are, not just what we do. It works like this:

- You have an experience
- Your experience triggers a memory
- Your memory triggers an emotional response landing somewhere on a spectrum from pleasant to unpleasant.
- A desire or craving arises in the form of an urge to take action or behave in ways that either bring about the cessation of unpleasant feelings or maintain pleasant feelings.
- You identify with this entire process from experience to feeling to craving to action. This circuit is your self-identity.

WAFFLES IN THE AFTERNOON: A CAUTIONARY TALE

Here's an example of how this idea of dependent origination can play out: You park your car on the wrong side of the street during a street cleaning day. In the morning, you bolt out of bed and run out to the street. Sure enough, there's that red envelope wedged beneath your windshield wiper. Recently your spouse has been criticizing you for being irresponsible and forgetting to do things around the house. For the last few weeks, you've been super stressed at work and you just don't have the space of mind or the energy for everything that needs to be done. But still, that ticket stings—it's your scarlet letter of shame. Proof that you are intrinsically absent minded. And now you're literally going to pay for it.

You've had this problem since you were a little kid. You used to daydream ... a lot ... and sometimes you'd forget err, neglect to do your homework, and your parents reprimanded you. Your parents and your spouse have put their fingers on a part of you that is fundamentally faulty, not good enough, broken. You are irresponsible and absent minded. It costs you, and it frustrates your spouse. What is your spouse going to say when she sees the ticket? It's going to confirm that you suck. You feel like crap about being this person who sucks. And you're frustrated because it feels like there's nothing you can do to not suck. So, with head hung low, you amble back inside and wander absentmindedly into the kitchen where you open the cupboard.

Mmm, there's that glossy blue king size box of frosted flakes with that jovial tiger on the front giving you a big thumbs up. He's been with you for decades now and never let you down. A jolt of pleasure ripples through your body. All of a sudden you feel a little lighter. You grab the biggest bowl from the cupboard and fill it to the brim with golden flakes encrusted with a pale shimmering coat of sugar. You drench it with near translucent non-fat milk—a healthy choice. You dig in. After a couple of bites, reality loses its edge. There's just that sweetness and subtle crunch. You forget about the ticket, your spouse, your parents. Your gaze softens as you stare out the window, but you're not really focusing on anything. Life is good. A little while later you step on the scale in the bathroom. Whoa, not good. You pinch your spare tire, check out your ass in the mirror. Yikes! Recently you've read somewhere that carbs make you fat, but what else is there to eat?

There's a list of things you need to do like mow the lawn and catch up on work, but you're tired and you just don't feel like it. It'd be nicer to just watch some TV while surfing the internet. You can't help thinking about all the things that need to get done, but you just don't have any energy or desire to do them. You pull up a delivery app on your phone and order waffles. Waffles in the afternoon.

YOU *ARE* YOUR CRAVINGS, BUT YOU DON'T HAVE TO BE!

This story demonstrates how your cravings, in this case for sugar, can distort and control the entire experience of what it is to be you. Yet, by practicing my keto way of life, we dismantle our most persistent and unhealthy cravings, fundamentally transforming our self-identities in profound ways. We discover that we are able to let go of habits that don't serve our highest and best good, and we are empowered with a new and profound ability to be present for challenges that in the past felt impossible to face and overcome. This is the foundations for fertility, both in our bodies and in our lives.

Fertile Presence

"Mindfulness is a way of befriending ourselves and our experience."
–Jon Kabat-Zinn

One of the most effective practices we can do to help ourselves grow our self-awareness and increase our fertility while cutting cravings is called ***mindfulness meditation***. Mindfulness is an essential part of my keto way of life, and it works by disrupting the automatic link between emotions and actions. When we practice mindfulness, a parking ticket in the morning won't result in doing nothing all day and eating waffles for lunch.

The model of dependent origination we've been working with to help us understand how we *are* our cravings was popularized by psychiatrist Dr. Jud Brewer, one of the world's leading mindfulness researchers. Dr. Brewer has created clinically proven mindfulness practices aimed at helping people overcome emotional eating. He's shown that mindful awareness is the tool that breaks the link between craving and action. So, what is mindfulness and how do we do it?

I define **mindfulness** as fully *being with* whatever is happening in the present moment without judgment and with a sense of gentleness, openness, and curiosity.

I define **meditation** as the simple exercise of becoming familiar with the qualities of mindfulness. Meditation is a way to train ourselves to be calmer, less reactive, and more compassionate in every area of our lives.

A TALE OF TWO BRAINS

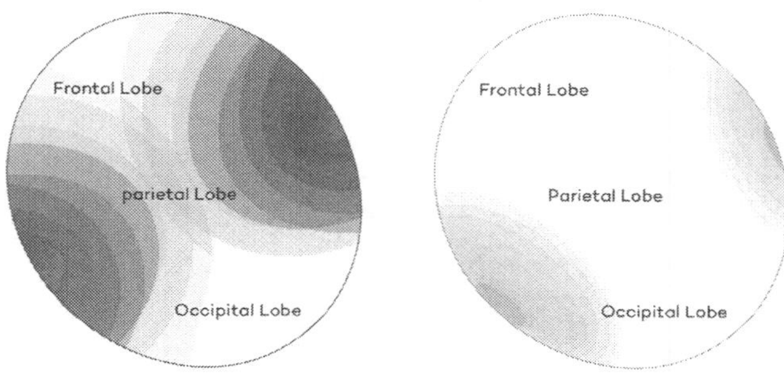

The image on the right shows a mind refined by mindfulness meditation. While the image on the left reveals an untrained mind wracked with the common mental chaos of distraction, stress, and anxiety. The mind on the right represents a person who is familiar with creating calm awareness. Though less activated, this person is actually more available to the splendor and beauty of a much broader spectrum of reality, even as their conscious state is a manifestation of the spiritual stillness that so many of us imagine we'll find at the top of a mountain.

Images like these come from a recent explosion of clinical trials aimed at discovering why and how mindfulness works and what it does for our brains and bodies. One of the most compelling insights we've discovered is that meditation decreases activity in areas of the brain associated with mind-wandering. This is important because when our minds are wandering, we're doing what psychologists call "self-referential" thinking. This means we're fantasizing about ourselves in the future and worrying about ourselves in the past. A recent study revealed that most of us are lost in mind wandering for a whopping 50% of our lives![vii] The problem with mind wandering is that it makes us self-conscious and judgmental in ways that take us out of the present moment and restricts our awareness of what is truly taking place in our lives and in the lives of others. Studies have also shown that mind wandering leads to depression, whereas a focused mind is a more positive mind.

Another study by Dr Amishi Jha reveals increased activity in the areas of the brain associated with cognitive control, which means we have more choice over what we focus on, how we react emotionally, and how we take action. Earlier research has shown that meditation boosts the left frontal activity of the brain, which is associated with positive mood, and decreased activity in the amygdala, a region related to stress and anxiety.

THE HAPPIEST PERSON IN THE WORLD

If you google "happiest person in the world," the first name that pops up is Matthieu Ricard, a seventy-year-old Tibetan Buddhist monk originally from France. His title as the happiest person came after Ricard took part in a twelve-year long brain study on meditation and compassion led by neuroscientist Richard Davidson at the University of Wisconsin.

With more than 10,000 hours of meditation under his belt, Ricard was the perfect subject to study to better understand the long-term effects of meditation. Researchers stuck 256 sensors to his head as he immersed himself in a form of compassion meditation popularly referred to as "loving kindness." The resulting brain scans showed levels of positively correlated brain waves that had never before been reported in the literature of neuroscience. His gamma waves read – .45 on a scale where – 0.3 is described as "beatific." His happiness scores were literally off the charts! The scans also showed extreme activity in his brain's left prefrontal cortex, the part of the brain that corresponds to positive emotions and thoughts.

By Ricard's own account, his 'happiness' comes from the way meditation trains him to think less about himself—i.e., self-referential mind wandering—and to feel more care and compassion for others. Ricard says. "It's simply that *me, me, me* all day long is very stuffy. And it's quite miserable, because you instrumentalize the whole world as a threat, or as a potential sort of interest [to yourself]."

Ricard counsels that happiness is not about accumulating an endless succession of experiences, rather happiness is a way of being. And that the deep, abiding happiness Ricard and other meditators cultivate is different than what most of consider as pleasures, which are transient and dependent on external factors. Happiness is a way of being present for every experience. Happiness is an orientation to life and not necessarily dependent or created by the content of life. The more we can cultivate this inner happiness, the healthier we become, both in our minds and bodies, and therefor the more fertile we become.

Mind-Body Medicine:

7 BENEFITS OF BRINGING MINDFULNESS INTO YOUR KETO WAY OF LIFE

In addition to pumping up our happiness scores, mindfulness has been clinically shown to benefit us in very specific psychological, emotional, and physical ways. These include:

1. STRESS & ANXIETY

Nearly 200 studies have confirmed that mindfulness practice has powerful positive effects on stress, negative moods, and anxiety. Though the right amount of pressure can be healthy and motivating, too much stress can be deadly. When we're stressed, our bodies produce a natural inflammation response, which can be helpful in short bursts, but when we're constantly stressed, our inflammation system never gets the chance to turn off. Chronic inflammation wreaks havoc on our bodies on a cellular level, resulting in chronic diseases and immune disorders. Combining the power of keto to reduce inflammation through metabolic processes with the power of mindfulness to reduce stress through our cognitive behaviors enhances the power of both diet and practice to bring our bodies back into balance.

2. EATING

Research on individuals without clinically diagnosed eating disorders found that mindfulness practice lead to a decline in binge eating as well as anxiety and depressive symptoms while increasing self-acceptance. These findings suggest that mindfulness breaks our craving cycles by reducing the power of negative emotions to drive our actions. This makes mindfulness practice a huge help when it comes to starting out on a keto diet. And once we've established our new eating practice, the combination of keto and mindfulness teams up to unlock us from limiting beliefs and harmful habits thereby empowering us to be present for the flourishing in our own lives in ways we have never before imagined.

3. DEPRESSION

Depression is one of the most common mental health issues in America and across the globe. Research shows that mindfulness meditation can be more powerful in alleviating depression than mainstream pharmaceutical treatments. As a doctor, I find that the fewer pills, pricks, and procedures a treatment entails, the better it is. The only thing you need to experience the positive effects of mindfulness is yourself.

Mindfulness gives us the direct experience of the transience of thoughts and emotions, freeing us from identifying with thoughts and feelings that bring us down. With mindfulness practice, we forge a perspective of wonder and compassion that we can apply towards all our thoughts and feelings, even those that we previously viewed as negative or too difficult to examine. In this way, mindfulness is extremely effective in helping us break the habits that can make beginning and maintaining a keto diet difficult. Additionally, there is a growing body of evidence linking depression and inflammation. And we know that keto works wonders in reducing inflammation.

4. COGNITIVE ABILITY

Research has found mindfulness practice produces significant improvements in critical cognitive skills after only four days of training for twenty minutes per day. Cognitive improvements are shown in the areas of sustained attention, increased working memory, and more skillful visuospatial processing. When you combine mindfulness with a ketogenic diet, you are maintaining and improving your cognitive functions through both your behavior and metabolic processes.

Researchers who conducted the study linking meditation with heightened visuospatial processing likened meditation to athletic training, stating that, "while engaging in intense physical activity, athletes often report entering a state similar to that achieved by meditators, often termed 'the zone.' In this state, athletes' physical abilities exceed their normal capacities: athletes exhibit enhanced speed in decision making, heightened attentional capabilities, and decreased fatigue. It is possible that the effects of meditation and 'the zone' are similar in some respects, although the effects of meditation are related to heightened mental capacities rather than heightened physical capacities."[viii]

5. IMMUNE FUNCTION

Researchers measured electrical activity in the brains of participants before and immediately after an 8-week meditation trial. After 8 weeks, both the meditators and control group (who did not meditate) were given an influenza vaccine. The group that had meditated produced significantly more antibodies than the non-meditators. The meditators also showed increased activity in the left frontal lobe of the brain. This research supports the power of mind-body medicine, where our thoughts and actions positively influence our wellbeing on a physiological level. Keto also supports the mind-body link from the direction of physiology to psychology. Other research has shown mindfulness practice to alleviate psoriasis, a skin disease that has a strong relationship with both emotional stress and physical inflammation.

6. RELATIONSHIPS

One of the most powerful effects of mindfulness is on our interpersonal relationships. Recent research has found that after just eight weeks of mindfulness practice participants showed a 50% increase in compassionate behaviors in real life situations compared to the control group that did not meditate. The key to increasing compassion comes from the self-awareness and non-judgmental acceptance at the heart of our practice. This leads to better communication of feelings while reducing social anxiety. Researchers have also found mindfulness to positively lead to greater relationship satisfaction by helping us be present for and communicate our feelings while reducing stress.

7. SLEEP

Mindfulness practices have been found to decrease the time it takes practitioners to fall asleep, while increasing total sleep time and quality. Often when we're lying awake trying to fall asleep, we're stuck in a cycle of reacting with frustration, worry, and pain to the thoughts and feelings churning through our minds. It's easy to get stuck in the self-referential thinking/craving cycle we discussed earlier. We can use mindfulness as a tool to change our relationship to our worries through creating acceptance and awareness that brings ease. Our practices change us from being merely reactive to being constructively responsive to our anxieties. With mindfulness, we step back and observe our thoughts and emotions without getting caught up in them. Combining mindfulness with keto will go even further by improving your slumber. Recent studies have shown that a keto diet increases high-quality REM sleep.

THREE TYPES OF MINDFULNESS PRACTICE

When you're just starting out on the journey of meditation, the word 'mindfulness' can be a little misleading. The 'mind' part of mindful doesn't just refer to the brain. Mind encompasses all of conscious experience. In my practice as a doctor over the last few decades, I see a relationship between mind and body that reflects the approach to meditation developed by ancient sages from over two thousand years ago: there is no divide between consciousness and our bodies. So, it's not surprising that there are various types of mindfulness practice aimed at honing our awareness towards both our physical and psychological experience.

Here's a brief summary of three fundamental types of mindfulness practice we can integrate into our keto way of life:

1. Awareness of breath: Pay attention to your breath, and when your mind wanders, gently shift it back to the awareness of your breath.
2. Loving-kindness: Think of someone in your life who genuinely and unconditionally wants the best for you. Alternately think of a time when you have wished well of others. Focus on this feeling and silently wish all beings wellness by repeating a few short phrases over and over. One common refrain is, "May all beings be happy, may all beings be healthy, may all beings be free from harm."
3. Choiceless awareness: Pay attention to anything that comes into your awareness, whether thought, emotion, or bodily sensation. Follow it until something else comes into your awareness without trying to chase after or hold onto it. When the next thing comes into your awareness, just pay attention to it until another things comes along.

Let Mindfulness *RAIN* Down

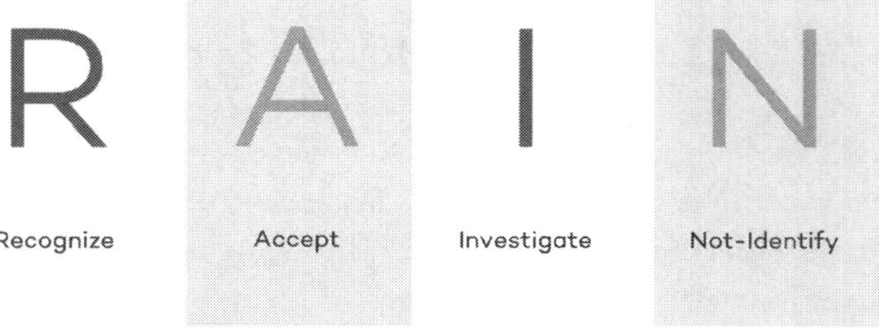

"Between the stimulus and the response there is a space, and in this space lies our power and our freedom."

-Victor Frankel

Mindfulness is about being in direct and vulnerable contact with ourselves. To be vulnerable in this way is to risk opening up to parts of ourselves that we avoid because they feel uncomfortable or scary. You could say that mindfulness training is actually vulnerability training. I'm reminded of a conversation I had with my friend Lena, a long-time psychologist. I asked her if she could identify one trait above all others that corresponded with psychological well-being. Without hesitating, she said, "Vulnerability." The more I deepened my own mindfulness practice, the more I understood the power of vulnerability to liberate us from our limitations and heal our physical and mental wounds.

Twenty years ago, mindfulness meditation teacher Michele McDonald came up with the easy to remember acronym *RAIN* to guide us towards greater vulnerability.

"Grace is courage under pressure"

-Ernest Hemmingway

R—Recognize your thoughts, feelings, and actions as they arise. Taking the frosted flakes story for example, this means noticing and naming emotions of frustration and loathing, feeling the physical manifestation of these emotions in the body as constriction in the neck and chest, and noticing the desire to binge on sugar, the feeling of relief, and the action of eating itself.

To recognize what's going on inside of ourselves in this way is like awakening from a trance. It's not easy to pay close attention to the critical inner-voice or to realize how incessant our self-doubt and painful feelings are. For many of us, recognizing what's going on is awakening to the war our thoughts, feelings, beliefs, and actions are waging on our bodies and spirits. Be brave and take heart! This is the first and most crucial step towards liberating yourself from your most persistent limitations.

"If it scares you, it might be a good thing to try."

-Seth Godin

A—Accept and allow your thoughts, feelings, and actions to simply be. This is a radical shift from our typical reactions to both pleasant and unpleasant experiences. With negative experiences, we tend towards self-judgement while attempting to dull or distract ourselves from the pain of the present moment. With positive experiences, we tend to become ego-inflated, causing us to lose sight of all the fortunate circumstances that colluded in our moment of satisfaction. We grow attached to the positive feelings, grasping ever tighter while getting bummed as they inevitably slip away and change. In both cases, we are unconsciously reacting to our experiences with attachment and aversion, causing us to lose sight, or never allowing ourselves to truly encounter the truth of the experience at the root of our reactions.

The emotional tone of acceptance is relaxation. It's an incredible relief to drop our resistance and just be with our feelings. In most instances, we discover that our contortions of fear and resistance were far more painful than the emotions we've been resisting. Being present with our emotions, no matter how seemingly negative, can be a euphoric release. Being with ourselves in this way is fundamentally about *being honest.* Honesty releases a tremendous amount of psychological pain and confusion.

One way to help ourselves encounter and be with difficult thoughts and feelings especially when they crop up around the challenge of becoming pregnant, is to repeat in whispers or say silently the word, YES. Saying yes activates the approach receptors in our brain, transforming our orientation from fear and defensiveness to openness, courage, and curiosity.

Instructions for living life:
Pay attention.
Be astonished.
Tell about it.

-Mary Oliver

I—Investigate with *curiosity* and compassion. Curiosity brings a natural desire towards honesty and truth, and therefore liberation. Curiosity has the power to liberate us from self-obsessive thought patterns, including comparisons and judgments that activate the whole cycle of attachment, aversion, and identification. Recent studies have shown that for even highly experienced meditators, bringing a tone of curiosity into an established practice can deepen its effects by dramatically reducing activity in regions of the brain associated with mind wandering and self-referential thinking. Curiosity aims our awareness towards what's happening in the present moment.

Investigating with curiosity means pausing to ask yourself *what is going on here? What does this feeling want from me? How does this feeling, thought, or belief manifest as a sensation in my body? What am I believing about myself or this situation that causes this feeling?* Curiosity expands our awareness by interrupting our habitual identification with our thoughts, feelings, and beliefs. There's a fundamental frequency shift when we switch from saying I am sad, or jealous, to saying hmm, that's interesting, there is sadness in me, jealousy in me, I wonder why this is? Or from saying I'm infertile, to saying it is difficult to conceive, I wonder what I can do to increase my fertility.

N—Natural awareness happens spontaneously when we Recognize, Accept, and Investigate our thoughts feelings and emotions. Though the first three steps of *RAIN* require intention and effort, the reward is the experience of natural awareness arising with an energy of its own in every aspect of our lives.

Natural awareness is often described as an openness and love of life. It happens when we've released our identification with our self-critical inner voice, and when we've made headway in understanding our limiting beliefs and the reactive actions that keep us in unhealthy cycles. Natural awareness arises with the realization that you are perfect just as you are, that there is nothing fundamentally wrong of flawed in you, and that you can accept your WHOLE self, even if you're struggling to conceive and give birth.

When you're first starting out on the path of mindfulness practice, each step of *RAIN* may feel like separate stages, yet you will soon find that when taken together, these stages describe the totality of mindfulness practice.

When we're being mindful, we are constantly recognizing, accepting, and investigating our thoughts, feelings, and behaviors within the space of loving awareness. There is no destination, nothing to achieve, no end goal. There is only a deepening awareness through the process.

Take this RAINS approach into any situation, from home life, to work, to quiet moments by yourself. Couple this process with gratitude and strengthen it with a keto diet, to transform your life and increase your fertility!

Here are a few guided practices that you can do anywhere—at home, at work, commuting etc. However, when just starting out and establishing your practice, it can be helpful to find a place that is relatively free from distractions. If you live with others, let them know that you don't want to be disturbed for the time you've allotted to your practice. With each of these techniques, you can begin by setting aside as little as 5 minutes a day, then gradually increasing by 5 minutes each week until you get to sessions of 20-30 minutes. If you're feeling motivated to create the most effective practice as quickly as possible, dive in for 20 – 30 minutes at a time.

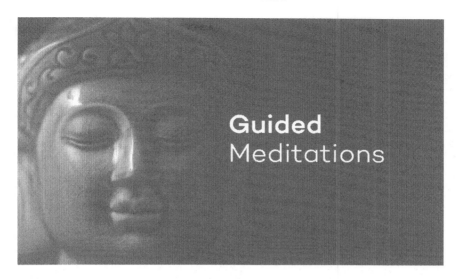

AWARENESS OF BREATH

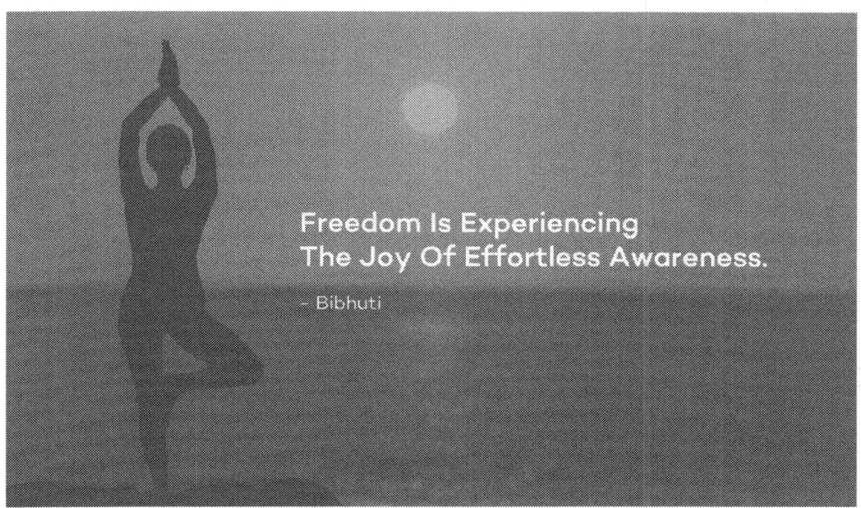

Freedom Is Experiencing
The Joy Of Effortless Awareness.

Find a comfortable seated position, or you can lie down if that's easier.
Gently shift your weight from side to side.
Feel the sensation of your body meeting the surface beneath you.
Feel the pressure of gravity gently holding you to the earth.

Feel the earth pressing back up against your body, supporting you, holding you.

Bring your awareness to your breath as it registers as a sensation in your nostrils.

Count ten breaths. Each inhale and exhale are a single breath.

Continue noticing your breath in your nostrils without counting.

Notice any thoughts.

When you notice a thought, label it by silently saying the word "thinking."

Gently and lovingly turn your awareness back to the sensation of your breath in your nostrils.

Notice how each inhale and each exhale are different from the last.

Each breath arising and passing away. Each breath unique.

Bring your awareness to your breath rising and falling in your chest.

When thoughts arise, gently and lovingly shift your awareness back to the sensation of your breath rising and falling in your chest.

Check in with your eyes—is there any tension there? Just notice the tension.

Gently shift your awareness back to your breath in your chest.

Now bring your awareness to your breath in your abdomen. The rise and fall of your stomach.

Each inhale and each exhale different than the last. Your body is constantly adjusting your oxygen levels. And you're just noticing the change. Noticing the rise and fall of your belly.

When thoughts arise, simply notice that you are thinking.

Notice how thoughts arise and pass away constantly, just as each breath arises and passes away.

Constantly changing.

Bring your awareness back to your breath rising and falling in your belly.

You are not chasing after or anticipating your thoughts, not pushing them away. They're just constantly erupting into the space of consciousness.

Gently shift your awareness back to the sensation of your breath rising and falling in your belly.

Now see if you can notice your breath registering in your whole body.
Your breath feeding every cell with oxygen.
It's a subtle sensation, but it's there.
Your breath filling and exiting your entire body.
Notice any tension in your jaw – it's natural for the jaw to get a little tighter as we concentrate.
Simply notice it. BE WITH IT.
Gently return your awareness to your breathing filling and emptying from your body.
When you're ready, wiggle your toes.
Wiggle your fingers.
Open your eyes (if you've closed them)
And surface into the world calm, refreshed, centered.

LOVING KINDNESS

Find a comfortable seated position, or you can lie down if that's easier.
Gently shift your weight from side to side.
Feel the sensation of your body meeting the surface beneath you.
Feel the pressure of gravity gently holding you to the earth.
Feel the earth pressing back up against your body, supporting you, holding you.
Close your eyes.
Think of someone who wishes you well, someone who loves you unconditionally, someone who wants to see you thrive. Maybe it's your mother, or your father, a teacher, or dear friend.
In your imagination, invite the loving person to sit before you, facing you.
Feel their love and care washing over you, saturating you.
Can you see this care flowing over and into you as a white light?
As you exhale, imagine this white light flowing from you back over the person.
Say to yourself, "May you be happy. May you be healthy. May you be free from harm."

Repeat this cycle-with each inhale, accept the white light flowing from them and saturating you.

With each exhale, watch the white light flowing from you back to them.

Repeat, "May you be happy. May you be healthy. May you be free from harm."

When you're ready to move on to your next guest, thank them for coming, let them go, and invite someone in your life toward whom you feel neutral.

Offer them this white light of compassion and wellbeing.

With each inhale, feel the light build in yourself, and with each exhale, watch the light wash over your guest.

Say to them, "May you be happy. May you be healthy. May you be free from harm."

When you're ready to move on, thank them for coming then let them go.

Think of someone for whom you have a complicated or fraught relationship. There's love and care, but it's not always clear because there may also be frustration and anger.

Invite this person before you. See them there facing you. Thank them for coming.

With each inhale feel the light build in yourself, and with each exhale, watch the light wash over your guest.

Say to them, "May you be happy. May you be healthy. May you be free from harm."

At first offering them this unconditional wish for wellbeing might be difficult. See if you can stick with it for six cycles.

Notice any tension in your body. Notice any release. Return to the person, to your breath, and the vision of white light flowing from you to them.

When you're ready to move on to the next stage, thank them for coming and let them go.

Now think of someone who you feel anger or antipathy towards, maybe even hatred.

Invite them before you into this space of compassion and wellbeing.

With each inhale, feel the light of loving kindness build in yourself.
With each exhale, watch the light wash over your guest.
Say to them, "May you be happy. May you be healthy. May you be free from harm."
Stick with it. Notice how the power of love and kindness in you is not affected by their presence. Notice them softening, getting clearer, releasing their guard, opening up to understanding.
When you feel ready to let them go, thank them for coming and watch them dissolve.
Now bring into your mind a picture of the earth.
With each inhale, feel the light of loving kindness build in yourself.
With each exhale, watch the light wash over the earth.
Say to yourself, "May all beings happy. May all beings be healthy. May all beings be from harm."
When you're ready, wiggle your toes, wiggle your fingers, slowly open your eyes, and return to the world filled with light and compassion.

CHOICELESS AWARENESS

Find a comfortable seated position, or you can lie down if that's easier.
Gently shift your weight from side to side.
Feel the sensation of your body meeting the surface beneath you.
Feel the pressure of gravity gently holding you to the earth.
Feel the earth pressing back up against your body, supporting you, holding you.
Pay attention to anything that comes into your awareness, whether thought, emotion, sound, or bodily sensation. Follow it until something else comes into your awareness, without trying to chase after or hold onto it.
When the next thing comes into your awareness, just pay attention to it until another thing comes along.
Notice how each aspect and each moment of reality is constantly arising, changing, and passing away.
There is nothing to grasp onto in the first place.
There is only the changing miracle of each and every moment.

Gaining Rather than Losing: Making the Transition to Keto

It's no coincidence that food and procreation are two of the most powerful forces motivating human beings. I often say that on the deepest most instinctive level, all people really want is to be *fed, made love to, put to bed, and have babies.* In my view these are 100% wholesome and natural desires. It's just that in modern society there are myriad forces out there manipulating these wholesome desires in unhealthy ways. As I've discussed earlier, the mainstream food industry is one of the most powerful and manipulative forces we have to contend with. The reason we're recommended to eat a varied diet is so that the food industry can sell us more stuff. We're not evolved for variety. We're not evolved to eat tons of grains and veggies. And we're certainly not evolved to eat the highly processed food that fills the aisles of your grocery store.

Yet we humans are genetically hard-wired to feel like we're in control of our lives, and to seek control when it feels like we don't have it. Saying, "I was brought up on pasta and it's a part of who I am," feels a lot better than saying, "I've been addicted to carbohydrates since I was kid and pasta is the way I get my fix."

As a fertility doctor, I have a front-row seat to these instincts on full display every day. The struggle to gain control over the ability to conceive and give birth is an incredibly powerful energy to be present for and to participate in. My proximity to the deepest realms of human desire has also revealed to me how we so often identify with our unhealthy habits and addictions. This reframe from addiction to identity gives us the illusion of control over the things that actually control and limit us. And it can be nearly impossible to give up these kinds of enabling illusions unless we're motivated by a clear vision of what we will gain by letting go of identities/habits that don't serve our highest and best good.

For many people the prospect of bringing new life into the world is the only force powerful enough to break this identity/addiction circuit. When it comes to my keto way of life, "new life" doesn't just mean babies—it means a more empowered, productive, awake, and connected version of *your own life!*

When preparing to make the transition to keto, it's important to remember that you're not losing anything by kicking carbs. Carbs are completely unnecessary; they are a sub-optimal energy source and the root of inflammation and disease. By following my keto way of life, you are activating all the disease fighting, energy generating, and clarity maintaining biological systems that your body has evolved over hundreds of thousands of years. You are increasing the quality of your life in the here and now, and you are extending the length and quality of your life into the future. You will feel more deeply connected to yourself and the people you love, and you'll have the energy and motivation to seek new challenges that expand your awareness and knowledge, while increasing your confidence and self-esteem.

Here are a few helpful tips to make the transition to the new you as smoothly and successfully as possible.

Pick a day to go keto and stick to it. Until then eat as you normally would:

If you try to cut-back on carbs before switching to keto, you'll just feel irritated and tired, and carbs will feel more precious than usual. The key is to make a clear transition to a fat-based diet. It may take a few days for your body to transition its metabolic systems, but if the food you are eating is meeting the macronutrient guidelines for your body weight and activity level, you should feel totally satiated from day one. In fact, you'll likely find that you want to eat less than the recommended portions. At first, I recommend fulfilling your daily calories, then later you can taper off.

Clean out your cupboards:
You are not giving anything up by cutting carbs, you're simply getting rid of something that makes you fat, sick, and infertile. Go through your cupboards and refrigerator and clean out everything that isn't specifically keto. Remember how easy it is to confuse free-will with habits and addiction. A good system will always be more effective than willpower, while saving you from the pitfalls of decision-fatigue—the tendency we have to lose our ability to resist temptations the more we are faced with them. After you clean out the carbs, it's important to stock your fridge and cupboards with ONLY keto specific foods. This way you'll avoid any lingering sense of deprivation. Keto is about abundance! We eat the most savory, nutrient packed foods that exist—bacon, eggs, butter, cream, beef, fatty fish, avocado, etc. When we stock up on these foods, we feel the primal satisfaction of having abundant access to the highest quality fuels that nature has created for our bodies and minds.

Carb withdrawal is no-big-deal and passes quickly:
When you cut the carbs, your body will go through a withdrawal period that feels like the onset of the flu. You may have body aches, dizziness, irritability and lethargy. For most people, this "keto flu" lasts between a few hours and a few days. It's totally natural and harmless, and there are steps you can take to make the transition easier.

- Stay hydrated by drinking plenty of water with added electrolytes. When your body switches into keto, the first thing it does is flush lots of salts. It's important to replenish your electrolytes with keto-specific nutritional supplements. You can find these online and at most grocery stores.
- Gentle exercise like a walk, bike ride, Tai Chi, or yoga, will help speed up the transition to keto by using up the glucose

stored in your bloodstream. Once the glucose is gone, your body switches to using fat for fuel.

- Remember that the discomfort you are feeling in the brief withdrawal period is the doorway to a new life of tremendous energy, clarity, and wellbeing.

Avoid alternative and artificial sweeteners:

There are no healthy substitutes for sugar. When we taste something sweet, even if it's sweetened with a "natural" alternative like stevia, our bodies react as if we're consuming calorie-rich sugar. When the sugar calories don't hit the bloodstream, our bodies crave sugar even more intensely. Artificial sweeteners like aspartame make us sick by fertilizing toxic intestinal flora and have been linked to stroke and heart-disease. So, stick to the program. Rather than easing the transition from carbs to keto, alternative and artificial sweeteners just prolong our addiction to carbs and make it more difficult to transition to a keto way of life.

Enjoy your keto way of life!

Make a daily practice of reflecting on all the energy and awareness you've unlocked by adopting a keto way of life. For most people, going keto spontaneously produces a deep abiding appreciation for the changes they've made. We can take inspiration from our own experiences by making a practice of verbalizing our gratitude and simply acknowledging the positive changes that are taking place in our lives either by speaking them aloud to ourselves or writing them down in a gratitude journal.

Part III: Fertile Plan

How to Keto

For most of you, keto is so radically different from your standard diet that it's easy to feel lost when figuring out how to shop, what to cook, and how to order when eating out. We have deep emotional attachments to the kinds of food we've been eating our whole lives, especially when we've been consuming a carb-heavy diet. Keto doesn't only mean switching to eating mostly fat—which is radical in its own right—it also means shedding a false belief system about nutrition that we've abided since we were children. While at the same time, keto calls on us to kick our emotional and biological addiction to sugar. I know it's not easy. Keto takes personal motivation, and it takes help. That's why this chapter is here.

As a rule of thumb when recommending keto to patients I suggest following what I call the B.E.B.B.I. Diet (pronounced "baby", because I am a fertility doctor after all) for its focus on bacon, eggs, butter, beef, and ice cream as its primary foods. I've incorporated these keto staples into meal plans and recipes for simplicity and ease. There are plenty of cookbooks out there with loads of elaborate keto twists on photogenic gourmet dishes. But for me, the beauty of keto is in how it simplifies our entire relationship to food, freeing up tremendous amounts of time and energy that we can put towards deeper relationships in all aspects of our lives, not only the things we eat. My aim with these guides is to get you comfortable with keto ASAP while helping you maintain consistency.

With that said, one of my favorite things about living a Ketogenic lifestyle is that I can eat healthfully and be satisfied too. There is no need to starve or feel like you're sacrificing your enjoyment of food and meals with friends and family. Nothing brings me greater joy than gathering with friends and family, sharing in each other's days and laughter while enjoying food that shows we care about ourselves just as much as each other.

Let's start with the exciting part—the foods you can eat freely, without restrictions or concerns.

Enjoy these foods!

Grass fed and wild animal sources

- Grass fed beef, lamb, goat, and venison
- Fish and seafood caught in the wild—not from the farm
- Pasteurized foods, including pork, poultry, eggs, gelatin, and ghee butter, all of which are high in Omega-3 Fatty Acid, which is good for us
- Offal, grass fed liver, heart, kidneys, and other organ meats
- Bacon—just pay attention to which kind you purchase. Uncured is best.

Healthy fats

- Saturated fats, which include: lard, tallow, chicken fat, duck fat, goose fat, clarified butter/ghee butter, coconut oil
- Monosaturated fats, which include avocado, macadamia, and olive oil
- Polyunsaturated Omega-3s, particularly ones found in animal sources
- Medium Chain Triglycerides (Refined coconut oil)

Vegetables that are non-starchy

- Leafy greens, including: bok choy, spinach, Swiss chard, lettuce, chard, collard greens, radicchio, endives, chives, etc.
- Cruciferous vegetables, which include: dark leaf kale, kohlrabi, and radishes

- Asparagus, cucumber, zucchini, celery stalk, and bamboo shoots

Fruits... this one may surprise you!

- Avocado—yes, that is the only one

Beverages and miscellaneous

- Water
- Coffee, either black or with coconut milk, ghee, MCT oils or organic cream
- Black or herbal teas
- Pork rinds, also known as cracklings, which can be used for breading instead of Panko crumbs or bread crumbs
- Lemon or lime juice and zest
- Natural proteins such as whey, egg white, and collagen, bone broth
- Condiments such as mayo, mustard, pesto, and pickles

Foods that can be the "exceptions" more than the "norm".

Fruits, mushrooms, and vegetables

- Low carb berries: raspberries, blackberries, strawberries
- Olives (both black and green)
- Coconut
- Rhubarb
- Certain root vegetables, including leeks, onions, garlic, mushrooms, pumpkin, parsley root, and spring onions
- Sea vegetables, which include kombu, okra, nori, bean sprouts, sugar snap peas, artichokes, sugar snap peas, and water chestnuts

Grain fed animal sources and full fat dairy

- Beef, poultry, ghee, and eggs

- Cottage cheese, cream, sour cream, and plain full-fat yogurt (avoid "low fat" as that usually means high sugar)

Seeds/nuts

- Macadamia nuts, pecans, almonds, walnuts, hazelnuts, Brazil nuts, and pine nuts flaxseed, pumpkin seeds, sesame seeds, sunflower seeds, and hemp seeds

Fermented products/soy products

- Non-GMO soy products including natto, tempeh, coconut aminos, and soy sauce
- Unprocessed green soybeans and black soybeans
- Fermented foods such as kimchi, sauerkraut, and kombucha

Condiments

- Thickening agents such as arrowroot powder
- Extra dark chocolate—70% up to 90%
- Cocoa and carob powder

Limited fruits, nuts, and vegetables with carbohydrates

- Fruits such as watermelon, cantaloupe, galia and honeydew melons
- Small amounts only of fruits such as apricots, peaches, nectarines, apples, grapefruit, kiwi, oranges, cherries, pears, and figs
- Nuts, including pistachios, cashews, and chestnuts
- Root vegetables, including: celery root, carrots, beetroots, parsnip, and sweet potatoes

Alcohol

- Dry red wines, including Cabernet Sauvignon, Merlot, Zinfandel, Pinot Noir, Syrah, Malbec, and Chianti
- Dry white wines, including Sauvignon Blanc, Pinot Grigio, Pinot Gris, Pinot Blanc, and Sémillon

Please note: alcohol works against weight loss and fertility goals

Meal Plans

For all of these meals I strongly recommend using the highest quality ingredients available to you. This is especially important when combining your keto diet with an intermittent feasting eating pattern. When fasting between meals, your body goes into a powerful regenerative state during which it lets old and damaged cells die off, while millions of new cells form.

It is *crucial* that you feed these new cells with clean fuels that you get from high quality foods like grass-fed and free-range meats, wild caught fish, unrefined oils, and organic eggs and dairy.

You'll notice that each day of the plan only has two main courses. This is to encourage you to eat less often, giving your body ample time to rest and digest. But have no fear! You'll quickly find that fat is far more satiating than carbohydrates, so you simply won't want to eat as much or as often. And to help you out, I've made the portions pretty big, so if you can't finish a meal in one sitting, feel free to save the rest for later. If you feel like you need more than two meals a day, especially when just starting out or when training, feel free to add in other recipes from different days. Bon appetite and bonne fertilité!

7 DAY MEAL PLAN

Day 1
Avocado Collagen Smoothie
Crème Fraiche Salmon

Day 2
Sausage Frittata with Spinach and Mushrooms
Garlic Butter Steak with Asparagus

Day 3
Eggs Scrambled with Cream Cheese, crème fraiche, avocado and pancetta.
Philly Cheesesteak Lettuce Wraps

Day 4
Deviled eggs with bacon and cheddar
Cast Iron Steak with Maitake and Blue Cheese

Day 5
Bacon and Eggs
Keto Pork Chops

Day 6
Stuffed Avocados with Bacon
Ribeye and Kohlrabi Stir Fry with Toasted Walnuts

Day 7
Sausage Egg Sandwich with Avocado
Keto Chili with Guacamole

DAY 1

AVOCADO SMOOTHIE

1 avocado, peeled and sliced
1 can full fat coconut milk
2 tablespoon collagen protein
2 tablespoons almond butter
1 tablespoon ghee
Juice from half a lime
1 cup ice

1. Place all ingredients in a blender and blend for 30 seconds, or until you reach your desired consistency. Pour into a glass and enjoy!

CRÈME FRAICHE DILL SALMON

1/4 cup butter, divided
Tablespoon dill, minced
½ pound salmon filet; dry, and room-temperature
1 teaspoon grated lemon zest
4 oz. crème fraiche
Salt and pepper to taste
Lemon wedges, for serving

1. Preheat your oven to 400F.
2. Mix the dill and lemon zest with the crème fraiche
3. Spread the crème fraiche evenly over the salmon.
4. Place the slices of butter on the crème fraiche.
5. Bake the salmon for appx 12 minutes, or until the fish is opaque and flakes easily with a fork.
6. Season with salt and pepper as needed, and serve warm with lemon wedges.

DAY 2

SAUSAGE FRITTATA WITH SPINACH

3 tablespoons ghee
1/2-pound ground sausage (Look for pork sausage with highest fat to protein ratio. Bratwurst is a good place to start, and as always organic and consciously raised is best. Avoid any sausages with preservatives)
2 cups fresh spinach, roughly chopped
5 eggs, beaten
2 oz. creme fraiche
Salt and pepper, to taste

1 tablespoon butter
1-pound asparagus, cleaned and trimmed
Half a lemon

1. Preheat your oven to 350F.
2. On medium-high heat, warm a 10" or 12" cast iron skillet. Add ghee and coat the pan as it melts.
3. Add the sausage and distribute evenly in the pan. Stir occasionally, allowing the meat to cook thoroughly if raw.
4. Once the sausage is cooked, add the spinach. Cook until spinach is slightly wilted, about 2-4 minutes. Sprinkle with salt and pepper.
5. Turn off the heat and distribute all the ingredients evenly within the pan. Then, pour the eggs into the pan. Place into the hot oven.
6. Cook for 20 minutes, or until the eggs are completely cooked through.
7. Season with salt and pepper to taste. Plate and serve with creme fraiche.

GARLIC BUTTER STEAK with ASPARAGUS

1 pounds boneless New York Strip or rib-eye steaks.
2 table spoons duck or beef tallow
1 cloves garlic, minced
1 sprig fresh thyme, finely chopped
2 tablespoons butter or tallow, for serving

1. Heat a large cast iron skillet over high heat for several minutes, until the pan begins to smoke.
2. Pat the steaks dry with a paper towel.
3. Add 1 tablespoon tallow to the pan and a brush the remaining tallow on the steak. Then generously season the steaks with salt and pepper.
4. Place steak in the hot pan and flip the steaks over every 30-45 seconds for around 6 minutes for a 1inch thick steak. Flipping them continuously will keep the steaks from developing a hard crust that can be carcinogenic.
5. Once the steaks are almost finished, reduce the heat to low and add butter, garlic, and herbs to the pan. Swirl around the pan to allow the butter to melt. Use a spoon to drizzle and baste the steaks until juicy on both sides. Flip the steaks after 20 seconds, to cook for 40 seconds with the butter.
6. Remove the steaks from the pan and cover loosely with foil. Allow the steaks to rest for 5 minutes before slicing.

FRIED ASPARAGUS

1. While steak is resting, heat the same pan over medium heat and melt 1 tablespoon of tallow. Add the trimmed asparagus and allow to heat and cook.
2. When the asparagus is hot, squeeze lemon juice over the pan and season with salt and pepper.

3. Cook until the asparagus softens and brightens in color, but still remains crunchy, about 3-4 minutes.
4. Serve alongside the steak and enjoy!

DAY 3

SCRAMBLED EGGS WITH CREAM CHEESE, CRÈME FRAICHE, PANCETTA, AND AVOCADO

4 Oz uncured diced pancetta
3 eggs
3 tablespoons cream cheese
1 tablespoon heavy cream
1 tablespoons butter
2 oz crème fraiche
½ Avocado

1. Whisk eggs together in a bowl. Add cream cheese and heavy cream and whisk until incorporated (chunks of cream cheese are OK).
2. Cook the pancetta in a cast-iron skillet until done.
3. Pour eggs into the pan and allow to sit, undisturbed, for about 20 seconds. Gently lift and fold the pancetta into the eggs.
4. Serve on a plate and top with crème fraiche and avocado.

BLUE CHEESE PHILLY CHEESESTEAK LETTUCE WRAPS

2 tablespoons butter.
4 large leaves of butter lettuce
1 tablespoon tallow
1 teaspoon dried oregano
Salt and pepper

1 pound skirt steak, thinly sliced
1 cup blue cheese
1 tablespoon freshly chopped parsley.

1. Add the steak to the hot pan in a single layer and season with salt and pepper. Stir until the steak is cooked
2. Sprinkle the blue cheese over the steak. Cover the skillet with a lid and turn off the heat, allowing the cheese to soften slightly. Remove from heat.
3. Arrange lettuce on a serving platter. Scoop the steak onto each piece of lettuce. Garnish with parsley and serve warm.

DAY 4

DEVILED EGGS WITH BACON AND CHEDDAR

6 large eggs, boiled and peeled
3 tablespoons organic olive oil or avocado based mayonnaise
1 teaspoon yellow mustard
1 teaspoon fresh dill weed
1/2 teaspoon salt
1/2 teaspoon pepper
1/2 cup grated cheddar cheese
4 slices bacon, cooked and crumbled

1. Slice the hard-boiled eggs in half and place yolks in a small mixing bowl. Set aside whites.
2. Add the mayonnaise, mustard, vinegar, dill, salt, and pepper to the mixing bowl with the yolks and stir well to combine.
3. Stir in the grated cheddar and crumbled bacon.
4. Spoon the filling into each of the egg whites.
5. Sprinkle with additional dill or bacon crumbles, as desired.

CAST IRON STEAK WITH MAITAKE AND BLUE CHEESE

1 large ribeye, at room temperature
3 tablespoons butter
1-3 sprigs of thyme
Salt and pepper
1/2 cup maitake mushrooms, whole or halved
1/4 cup blue cheese

1. Pat the steak dry with a paper towel and season liberally with salt and pepper.
2. Heat a large cast iron skillet over high heat.
3. Sear steaks for 1 minute on each side, then reduce the heat to medium high.
4. Add butter and thyme and distribute evenly around the pan.
5. Flip the steak every 30 seconds for 10 minutes, or until the steak is cooked to your desired level of doneness. Use a spoon to baste the steak with each flip.
6. When done, place the steak on a cutting board or platter and loosely cover with tinfoil. Allow the steaks to rest for five minutes before cutting or serving.
7. While steak rests, add the maitake mushrooms to the pan. Coat in the remaining butter and cook until softened and brown.
8. Serve mushrooms alongside steak and sprinkle liberally with the blue cheese.

DAY 5

BACON AND EGGS

3 large eggs
1/3 cup heavy whipping cream
1 tablespoon butter
4 slices of bacon
Salt and pepper

1. Preheat oven to 350F.
2. Lay the bacon on a cookie sheet and bake for 10-15 minutes, until cooked to your liking.
3. In a bowl, add eggs and cream and whisk lightly.
4. Heat a large pan to medium-low and add the butter.
5. Once the butter has melted, add the eggs. Allow them to sit, untouched, for thirty seconds.
6. Then, gently lift and fold the eggs to stir until they are just cooked. Add salt and pepper.
7. Place eggs and bacon on a plate and enjoy warm.

KETO PORK CHOPS

1-pound bone-in-center pork chop
Salt and pepper
1 clove garlic
2 tablespoons butter
1 tablespoon tallow
1 tablespoon apple cider vinegar
1 tablespoon ghee

1. Season the pork chops with salt and pepper.
2. Heat a large cast iron skillet over high heat. When the pan is very hot, add the ghee and then the pork. Turn the heat down slightly so you do not burn the ghee. Sear the pork chops for 5-7 minutes until the bottom is very brown.
3. Flip the prod and add the garlic and butter. When the butter is melted, tilt the pan to distribute evenly throughout the pan. Use a spoon to baste the pork chops in butter.
4. After 2-3 minutes, remove the cooked pork chops from the pan.
5. Then, add in the apple cider vinegar to the pan. This releases the browned bits from the bottom of the pan. Scape them off with a wooden spoon. Return the chops to the pan and cover with the sauce, add tallow. Serve warm.

DAY 6

BACON STUFFED AVOCADOS

6 slices bacon
2 avocados, halved and pits removed
1/2 lemon
1 green onions, trimmed and sliced
1/2 cup organic sour cream
1 tablespoon chopped parsley, optional
Salt and pepper

1/4 cup olive oil
1/4 cup fresh lemon juice
1 clove garlic, minced
Salt and pepper

1. Preheat your oven to 350°. Bake the bacon to your desired crispness, about 10-15 minutes, on a baking sheet. When the bacon is cool, crumble it into a large bowl.
2. Cut the avocados, remove the pits, and scoop out the flesh. Save the avocado peels.
3. Dice the avocados and add them to the bowl with the bacon.
4. Squeeze lemon juice over the diced avocados and empty peels. This will prevent browning.
5. Add the diced sour cream to the bowl, and mix. Season with salt and pepper to taste.
6. To make the lemon dressing, whisk together all the ingredients in a small bowl, adjusting the seasonings to taste.
7. Pour the dressing over the salad and stir gently.
8. With a spoon, scoop out the avocado mixture and fill the empty avocado shells. Add additional sour cream, as desired.
9. Garnish with sliced green onions, parsley, and fresh black pepper. Enjoy!

RIBEYE AND KHOLRABI STIR FRY WITH TOASTED WALNUTS

12 ounces ribeye steak
3 ounces broccoli
5 ounces butter, divided
Salt and pepper
2 tablespoon toasted walnuts, roughly chopped

1. Pat the steak dry with a paper towel, then thinly slice. Chop the onion and broccoli.
2. Heat half of the butter in a frying pan or a wok. Add the meat and cook for 9 minutes, flipping every 30 seconds to avoid charring.
3. Season with salt and pepper and remove from the pan and set aside, covered.
4. Add the remaining butter and cook the kohlrabi in the same pan. Just when the vegetables are softened and hot, add the soy sauce and stir to coat the vegetables.
5. Return the meat back to the pan, along with the walnuts, and stir to combine.
6. Season to taste and serve warm.

DAY 7

SAUSAGE EGG SANDWICH WITH AVOCADO

2 sausage patties
1-2 eggs, room temperature
3 tablespoons heavy cream
1 tablespoon cream cheese, room temperature
2-3 tablespoons cheddar cheese
1/4 avocado, sliced
Salt and pepper, to taste

1. In a large pan, cook the sausage per instructions on the package and set aside.
2. In a small bowl, combine cream cheese and cheddar cheese and quickly stir with a fork to break up the cream cheese a bit.
3. In another bowl, gently whisk eggs and cream. Add salt and pepper.
4. Cook eggs in the same pan as the sausage. Making a small omelet that will fit nicely on the sausage patties, add cheese mixture.
5. Assemble the sandwich, placing the omelet on one of the sausage patties, topping with avocado and then the second sausage patty. Enjoy warm.

TUNA PATTIES

2 5-ounce cans sustainable tuna, drained
1/6 cup almond flour
1 green onion, chopped white and light green parts only
1 tbsp chopped fresh dill
1 tbsp lemon zest
3/4 tsp salt
1/2 tsp pepper
1/4 cup organic olive oil or avocado oil-based mayonnaise
1 large egg
1 tbsp freshly squeezed lemon juice
1 tbsp avocado oil

1. Drain the tuna well.
2. Use a low carb binder such as almond flour or coconut flour, to help the patties hold their shape.
3. Add mayo.
4. Form by hand into firm 3/4-inch-thick 3-inch diameter patties.
5. Fry in a non-stick skillet. Flipping carefully.
6. Serve with toppings like Garlic Aioli Mayo and capers.

KETO CROWD PLEASERS

These easy-to-make recipes can be substituted into your weekly meal plan for breakfast, lunch, or dinner. I find these recipes to be really fun to make and they're fantastic when cooking for others who are unfamiliar with keto, or when you need to bring something to a potluck or dinner party that you and everyone else will enjoy.

BACON AVOCADO AND BAKED EGG NEST

1 large avocado
2 eggs
1 strip bacon cooked
(multiply each ingredient by number of guests you are cooking for)

1. Preheat the oven to 400 degrees.
2. Cut avocado in half and remove pit.
3. Using a spoon, widen the hole of each half by removing about a teaspoon of flesh.
4. Place your avocados into a baking dish
5. Crack eggs into each hole, sprinkle with salt and pepper.
6. Bake for 15-20 minutes.
7. Chop bacon into small pieces and sprinkle on top of eggy avocados.

KETO TUNA MELT

(Serves 4)

Tuna mix:
1 cup mayonnaise or sour cream
4 celery stalks
½ cup dill pickles, chopped
8 oz. tuna in olive oil

1 tsp lemon juice
1 garlic clove, minced
salt and pepper, to taste

Oopsie bread:
3 eggs
4½ oz. cream cheese
1 pinch salt
½ tbsp ground psyllium husk powder
½ tsp baking powder

Topping:
⅔ lb. shredded cheese
¼ tsp cayenne pepper or paprika powder
For serving
5 oz. leafy greens
olive oil

1. Preheat the oven to 300°F (150°C).
2. Separate the egg yolks into one bowl and the egg whites into another.
3. Whip egg whites together with salt until very stiff. You should be able to turn the bowl over without the egg whites moving.
4. Mix the egg yolks and the cream cheese well. Add the psyllium seed husk and baking powder.
5. Gently fold the egg whites into the egg yolk mix – keep the air in the egg whites as best you can.
6. Make 4-6 oopsies on a parchment-lined baking tray.
7. Bake in the middle of the oven for about 25 minutes or until they turn golden.

Tuna mix and serving

1. Preheat the oven to 350°F (175°C).
2. Mix the salad ingredients well.

3. Place the bread slices on a baking sheet lined with parchment paper. Spread the tuna mix on the bread and sprinkle cheese on top.
4. Add some paprika powder or cayenne pepper.
5. Bake in oven until the cheese begins to crisp—about 15 minutes.
6. Serve the sandwich with some leafy greens like parsley or arugula, drizzled with olive oil.

KETO BACON SUSHI

6 slices bacon, halved
2 Persian cucumbers, thinly sliced
2 medium carrots, thinly sliced
1 avocado, sliced
4 oz. cream cheese, softened
Sesame seeds, for garnish

1. Preheat oven to 400°.
2. Line a baking sheet with aluminum foil.
3. Lay bacon halves in an even layer and bake until slightly crisp but still pliable, 11 to 13 minutes.
4. Cut cucumbers, carrots, and avocado into sections roughly the width of the bacon.
5. When bacon is cool enough to touch, spread an even layer of cream cheese on each slice.
6. Divide vegetables evenly between the bacon and place on one end.
7. Roll up vegetables tightly.
8. Garnish with sesame seeds and serve.

KETO TACO CUPS

2 c. shredded cheddar
1 tbsp. extra-virgin olive oil or ghee

1 small onion, chopped
3 cloves garlic, minced
1 lb. ground beef
1 tsp. chili powder
1/2 tsp. ground cumin
1/2 tsp. paprika
Kosher salt
Freshly ground black pepper
Sour cream, for serving
1 Diced avocado
Freshly chopped cilantro

1. Preheat oven to 375°.
2. Line a large baking sheet with parchment paper.
3. Spoon about 2 tablespoons cheddar a few inches apart. Bake until bubbly and edges are beginning to turn golden, about 6 minutes.
4. Let cool on baking sheet for a minute.
5. Grease bottom of muffin tin with butter or ghee.
6. Using care, pick up melted cheese slices and place on bottom of muffin tin.
7. Mold the cheese around the tin.
8. In a large skillet over medium heat, heat ghee or olive oil.
9. Add onion and cook until softened, about 5 minutes.
10. Stir in garlic, then add ground beef. Cook until beef is no longer pink, about 6 minutes, then drain fat.
11. Return meat to skillet and lightly season with chili powder, cumin, paprika, salt, and pepper
12. Transfer cheese cups to a serving platter. Fill with cooked ground beef and top with sour cream, avocado, cilantro.

KETO QUESIDILLAS

1 tbsp extra-virgin olive oil or ghee

1 bell pepper, sliced
1/2 yellow onion, sliced
1/2 tsp. chili powder
Kosher salt
Freshly ground black pepper
3 c. shredded Monterey Jack
3 c. shredded cheddar
4 c. shredded chicken
1 avocado, thinly sliced
1 green onion, thinly sliced
½ cup crème fraiche or sour cream

1. Preheat oven to 400° and line two medium baking sheets with parchment paper.
2. In a medium skillet over medium-high heat, heat olive oil or ghee.
3. Add pepper and onion and season with chili powder, salt, and pepper. Cook until soft, 5 minutes. Transfer to a plate.
4. In a medium bowl, stir together cheeses. Add 1 1/2 cups of cheese mixture into the center of both prepared baking sheets. Spread into an even layer and shape into a circle, the size of a flour tortilla.
5. Bake cheeses until melty and slightly golden around the edge, 8 to 10 minutes.
6. Add onion-pepper mixture, shredded chicken, and avocado slices to one half of each.
7. Let cool slightly, then use the parchment paper and a small spatula to gently lift and fold one side of the cheese "tortilla" over the side with the fillings.
8. Return to oven to heat, 3 to 4 minutes more.
9. Repeat to make 2 more quesadillas.
10. Cut each quesadilla into quarters. Garnish with green onion and plenty of sour cream before serving.

TO TIDE YOU OVER

I get it! Eating only twice a day or within a restricted time period can be tough at first. These quick and easy fat-filled recipes will give you the fuel to make it across the finish line—and take a few more laps!

NO BAKE CACAO FAT BOMBS

1 cup nut butter of choice, or coconut butter
1/2 cup cocoa or cacao powder
1/2 cup melted coconut oil
optional, I like to add 1/8 tsp salt

Stir all ingredients together until smooth. If too dry (depending on the nut butter you use), add additional coconut oil if needed. Pour into a small container, ice cube trays, or candy molds. Freeze to set. Coconut oil softens at room temp so it's best to store these in the freezer or fridge.

BACON, CHIVE AND CHEDDAR MUG CAKE

A serving is 573 calories with 31.3g of fat, 0 g of proteins, and 4.3g net carbohydrates.
Serves 1-2 people

1 large egg
Pinch of salt
3 Tbsp almond flour
2 slices of cooked, chopped bacon
1 Tbsp of cheddar cheese
1 Tbsp of chopped chive
2 Tbsp of grass-fed butter
1/2 tsp of akin powder
1 Tbsp of shredded white cheddar

1/4 tsp of non-salt blend of seasoning (your favorite)

Combine all ingredients in bowl aside from bacon and chives. Mix thoroughly and then add the bacon in, mix again, and then pour into a ramekin or a mug. Microwave on high for 2 minutes (depends on microwave), and then top with chives and serve.

KETO ROASTED GARLIC CHIPOTLE AIOLI

At 76 calories, it has only 8.2g of fat, .4g of protein, and .4 net carbohydrates.
Makes 36 servings
1 Tbsp roasted garlic
1/4 cup sour cream
2 tsp lemon juice
1/4 tsp chipotle powder
1/2 cup olive oil
2 large egg yolks
1 tsp Dijon mustard
Pinch of salt and black pepper

If eggs are cold, place them in warm water for one minute to bring them to room temperature. Put the yolks into a food processor, along with the mustard, lemon juice, and garlic. Blend the mixture together while adding the oil. Afterward, salt and pepper to taste and blend again until mixture is thoroughly combined. Stir in the chipotle and sour cream, and mix again. Chill and serve!

KETO RASPBERRY LEMON POPS

At 151 calories with 16g of fat, .5g of protein, and only .2 net carbohydrates, these are treats that hit the spot!
Serves 6
1 cup of raspberries
1/4 cup of coconut oil

1/4 cup of sour cream
1/2 tsp of Guar gum
1/2 lemon, juiced
1 cup of coconut milk
1/4 cup of heavy cream
20 drops of liquid Stevia

Put all ingredients into a blender and pulse until mixture is thoroughly combined. Afterward, pour mixture through a strainer and pour into popsicle molds. Let them freeze for 2 hours or longer. Then enjoy!

AVOCADO LIME SORBET

180 calories of deliciousness! With 16g of fat, 2g of protein, and net carbohydrates of only 3.5, this is a fantastic dessert or treat.
Serves 4

2 avocados
2 limes, squeezed and zested
1/4 tsp liquid Stevia
1/4 cup of Erythritol powder
1/4 cup of cilantro
1 cup of coconut milk

Remove the seed and peel it from the avocados, and then cut into thin slices. Place the slices on a baking sheet and squeeze 1 lime over the avocados, freeze for 3 hours or more. Then, add milk, lime zest, and Erythritol to a saucepan and boil over, until about 1/4 of the liquid has evaporated. Remove from heat and put into the freezer to cool mixture, until mixture has thickened. Next, you'll chop cilantro and add to a food processor, along with the frozen avocados and remaining lime juice. Chop until chunky and then put Stevia and coconut milk in. Blend to desired consistency and serve, or pour into small containers and freeze until ready to use.

VEGETARIAN MEAL PLAN

Day 1
Avocado Smoothie
Endive, Walnut, and Blue Cheese Salad with Soft-Boiled Egg

Day 2
Egg and Cream Cheese Scramble
Zucchini Lasagna

Day 3
Omelet with Spinach and Cream Cheese
Coconut Stir-Fried Vegetables with Cauliflower Rice

Day 4
Cashew Smoothie
Vegetarian Keto Burritos

Day 5
Brussel Sprout Hash with Fried Eggs
Coconut Curry with Cauliflower Rice

Day 6
Vanilla Overnight "Oats"
Spinach and Artichoke Egg Casserole

Day 7
Keto Scrambled Eggs
Zucchini Noodles with Avocado Cream

DAY 1

AVOCADO SMOOTHIE

1/2 avocado, peeled and sliced

1/2 can full fat coconut milk
1/2 cup almond milk
2 tablespoons almond butter
1 tablespoon unrefined coconut oil
Juice from half a lime
1 teaspoon Spirulina (optional)
1 cup ice (or more for a thicker smoothie

1. Place all ingredients in a blender and blend for 15 seconds, or until you reach your desired consistency. Pour into a glass and enjoy!

ENDIVE, WALNUT, AND BLUE CHEESE SALAD WITH SOFT-BOILED EGG

4-6 endives, thinly chopped
1 cup toasted walnuts, roughly chopped
1/2 cup blue cheese
3 tablespoons olive oil
3 tablespoons champagne vinegar
1 teaspoon lemon juice
3 eggs, soft boiled, cooled, and roughly chopped
Salt and pepper, to taste

1. Place endives and walnuts in a medium bowl.
2. In a small bowl, whisk together the oil, vinegar, lemon juice, and salt and pepper. Pour over endives and walnuts and stir to combine.
3. Add the blue cheese and chopped egg and gently stir until everything is just mixed.

DAY 2

EGG, RED PEPPER, AND CREAM CHEESE SCRAMBLE

4 eggs
1 small red bell pepper
3 tablespoons cream cheese
1 tablespoon heavy cream
1 tablespoons butter
1-2 tablespoons chives, finely chopped

1. Whisk the eggs together in a bowl. Add cream cheese and heavy cream and whisk until incorporated (small chunks of cream cheese are OK).
2. Melt the butter in a cast-iron skillet on medium heat. Add the red peppers and cook for about 2 minutes, until softened. Season with salt and pepper. Add the chives and cook for another minute.
3. Slowly, pour the eggs into the pan and allow to sit, undisturbed, for about 30 seconds. Then, gently lift and fold the eggs to stir them until they are just cooked. Turn off the heat.
4. Serve and enjoy warm.

ZUCCHINI LASAGNA

Sauce
1 tablespoon olive oil
1 large onion
4 garlic cloves, minced
2 bay leaves
1 teaspoon cinnamon
1 teaspoon dried oregano
1 28 ounce can crushed tomatoes

Lasagna
3 large zucchini
3-4 cups mozzarella cheese, shredded
2 cups mushroom slices
1 1/2 cups ricotta cheese
1/2 cup parmesan cheese
1 tablespoon parsley, for garnish

1. Make the sauce. Add the olive oil to a large skillet over medium-high heat. Add the onion and cook for 2 minutes, until onion is soft. Add the garlic, bay leaves, oregano, and pepper. Stir until spices bloom. Add crushed tomatoes, stir, and simmer for 10 to 15 minutes.
2. While the sauce is simmering, prepare the zucchini. Slice the zucchini so they are 1/8 of an inch thick.
3. Preheat the oven to 375F.
4. Using a 9x13 inch baking dish, assemble a layer of zucchini in the bottom of the dish. Top with mozzarella and mushroom slices. Then add a layer of sauce, followed by dollops of ricotta cheese.
5. Repeat this layer 3 times. Top with shredded mozzarella cheese. Sprinkle parmesan over the top.
6. Bake for 40 to 50 minutes. The top should be golden and the cheese should bubble.
7. Allow the lasagna to sit and cool for about 15 minutes before slicing and serving. Garnish with parsley. Serve warm and enjoy.

DAY 3

OMELET WITH SPINACH AND CREAM CHEESE

1 tablespoon butter
4 eggs, room temperature
3 tablespoons heavy cream

2 tablespoon cream cheese, room temperature
2-3 tablespoons cheddar cheese, shredded
1 cup spinach
Salt and pepper, to taste

1. In a small bowl, combine cream cheese and cheddar cheese and quickly stir with a fork to break up the cream cheese a bit.
2. In another bowl, gently whisk eggs and cream. Add salt and pepper.
3. Melt butter in a medium sized pan over medium high heat. Add eggs and do not touch but allow the bottom to cook. After a few minutes, the top will begin to congeal. Add the cheese mixture and the spinach, and close the omelet. Fold one or two times, to your preference.
4. When the middle has set, remove from the heat and sprinkle with salt and pepper, to taste. Serve warm and enjoy.

COCONUT STIR-FRIED VEGETABLES WITH CAULIFLOWER RICE

3 cups cauliflower florets
2 cups broccoli florets
1 cup baby carrots
2 tablespoons toasted sesame seed oil
1/3 cup red onion, minced
1 teaspoon freshly grated ginger
2 garlic cloves, minced
1 cup full-fat coconut milk
2 tablespoons soy sauce
Salt and pepper, to taste
2 tablespoons unrefined coconut oil
1/4 cup unsweetened large coconut flakes, toasted

1. Place the cauliflower in the container of a food processor. Chop until it is about the same size as rice. Set aside.

2. In a large pan or wok, heat the sesame oil and then fry the broccoli and carrots for about 4-5 minutes. Add the onions and fry for 2 more minutes or so, until the vegetables are crisp and tender. Transfer the vegetables to a bowl and cover loosely with a lid or foil to keep warm.
3. In the same pan, add the ginger and garlic. Cook for 30 seconds, will constantly stirring.
4. Add the coconut milk, soy sauce, salt and pepper. Bring to a boil, then reduce the heat and simmer, uncovered, for 5 minutes. You want the sauce to thicken slightly.
5. In another large skillet, heat the coconut oil over medium heat. Add the cauliflower rice and season with salt and pepper. Cook while stirring frequently, for about 5 minutes. The cauliflower should be tender and just beginning to brown.
6. Return the vegetables to the pan with the sauce. Cook and stir for 1 minute to heat the vegetables through. Turn off the heat.
7. Scoop cauliflower rice onto plates and top with vegetables and sauce. Serve warm and enjoy.

DAY 4

CASHEW SMOOTHIE

2/3 cup unsweetened cashew milk (or other milk of choice)
3 tablespoons natural cashew butter
2 tablespoons hemp hearts
2 tablespoons chia seeds
2 tablespoons coconut oil
1 cup fresh spinach
1/2 cup frozen strawberries
1 cup ice

1. Place all ingredients into a blender and blend for 15 seconds, or until you reach your desired consistency. For a thicker consistency, add more ice or frozen strawberries. Enjoy!

VEGETARIAN KETO BURRITOS

6 homemade Keto tortillas*
1 small red pepper, sliced
1 small yellow pepper, sliced
1 medium red onion, sliced
1 large zucchini, chopped
2 tablespoons olive oil
1/4 teaspoon cumin
1 teaspoon paprika
1 cup chopped kale, packed
3 cups cauliflower florets
3 tablespoons unrefined coconut oil, melted
1 cup cheddar cheese, grated
1 cup sour cream
2 tablespoons chopped cilantro (optional)
Juice from 1/2 a lime
Salt and pepper, to taste

Tortillas
1 cup almond flour
3/4 cup packed cup flax meal
1/4 cup coconut flour
2 tablespoons whole psyllium husks
2 tablespoons ground chia seeds
1 teaspoon salt
1 cup water
2 tablespoons lard, or olive oil, or ghee

1. Prepare the keto tortillas.

2. Preheat the oven to 375F. Chop the peppers, onion, and zucchini into Small chunks. Toss with olive oil, cumin, paprika, and generous amount of salt and pepper. Roast in the oven for about 20 minutes, until vegetables are cooked and soft.
3. Place the cauliflower florets in a food processor and blitz until it resembles a rice consistency. Cook on the stove with a dash of water. Then, strain out the excess water and place in a bowl with the coconut oil and a pinch of salt.
4. When the vegetables are cooked, roughly chop the kale and massage gently to soften it. Mix it in with the other vegetables to incorporate all the flavors. Cook all the vegetables together for 2-4 more minutes. Remove from the oven.
5. Stuff each tortilla with cauliflower rice, roasted vegetables, grated cheese, and top with a good dollop of sour cream, lime juice, cilantro garnish, and fresh ground pepper.

1. To make the tortillas, place all of the dry ingredients in a bowl.
2. Add the water and mix well with your hands – use more water *only* if you need to. Then allow the dough to rest in plastic wrap in the refrigerator for at least an hour.
3. When rested, cut the dough into 6 equal pieces. Place a piece of the dough between two pieces of parchment paper and roll with a rolling pin until it is very thin. Use an 8" bowl or pot lid to cut out a large circle.
4. Repeat until you have six tortillas
5. Then, preheat a large cast-iron pan with 1 tablespoon lard. Place the tortillas, one at a time, in the pan and cook over medium heat for 1-2 minutes, until the tortilla is lightly browned. Flip and cook for 30 – 60 more seconds. Add more lard as needed.

DAY 5

BRUSSELS SPROUT HASH WITH EGGS AND CHEDDAR

2 tablespoons butter

2 tablespoon olive oil
1 tablespoon balsamic vinegar
2 garlic cloves, minced
Salt and pepper
2 pounds Brussels sprouts, halved

4 large eggs
1/4 cup grated cheddar
Salt and pepper
2 tablespoons freshly chopped chives
Sour cream

1. Preheat the oven to 400F. Lightly oil a baking sheet with nonstick spray.
2. In a small bowl, whisk together the balsamic vinegar and olive oil. Season with salt and pepper.
3. Place Brussels sprouts in a single layer onto the prepared baking sheet. Cover in the balsamic vinegar mixture.
4. Place in the oven and bake for 10-12 minutes.
5. Remove from the oven and create 4 wells in the pan. Gently crack the eggs in each well, doing your best to keep the yolk intact.
6. Sprinkle eggs with cheddar. Season with salt and pepper to taste.
7. Return the pan to the oven and bake until the egg whites have set, an additional 8-10 minutes.
8. Garnish with chives and sour cream, if desired, and serve warm.

TOFU COCONUT CURRY WITH CAULIFLOWER RICE

1 1/2 pounds tofu
2 Tablespoons unrefined coconut oil
1 1/4 cup full fat coconut milk
4 teaspoons red curry paste

1/3 cup red onion, diced
Olive oil
Salt and pepper
Fresh cilantro, chopped
3 cups cauliflower florets

1. Preheat oven to 400F.
2. Chop the tofu into small cubes and marinate in 2 teaspoons of the red curry paste. Set aside in the refrigerator for 20 minutes.
3. Place coconut oil in a large cast-iron skilled and set on medium heat. Add onions and 2 teaspoons of red curry paste. Cook the onions in the paste for 5 minutes until soft.
4. Add the tofu and do not stir – searing the tofu to a dark golden brown will bring out more flavor.
5. When the tofu has browned, reduce the heat and add the coconut milk. Bring to a simmer and turn off the heat.
6. Place the entire skillet in the oven and bake for 12 to 15 minutes.
7. To make the cauliflower rice, blitz 3 cups of cauliflower florets in a food processor. Cook on the stovetop with a dash of water, then strain and dress as desired.
8. Scoop rice into bowls and top with tofu curry sauce. Garnish with fresh cilantro. Enjoy!

DAY 6

VANILLA OVERNIGHT "OATS"

1/3 cup hemp hearts
1/3 cup unsweetened almond milk (or other milk of choice)
2 tablespoons almond butter
1 tablespoon unrefined coconut oil
2 teaspoons chia seeds
1 teaspoon vanilla extract
Vanilla seeds from 1/2 of a vanilla bean (optional)
Nuts and seeds, fruit and berries (optional)

1. Mix all the ingredients together in a large mason jar.
2. Refrigerate for 1 hour, or overnight.
3. Garnish with nuts, seeds, berries, or fruit.

SPINACH AND ARTICHOKE EGG CASEROLE

16 large eggs
1/4 cup heavy cream
1 can artichoke hearts, drained
5 cups fresh spinach
1 cup cheddar cheese, grated
1/2 cup parmesan cheese
1/2 cup ricotta cheese
1/2 cup onion, chopped
2 cloves garlic, minced
1 teaspoon salt
1/2 teaspoon dried thyme
Salt and pepper, to taste

1. Preheat the oven to 350F. Spray a 9x13" baking dish with nonstick cooking spray.
2. Place the eggs and heavy cream in a medium bowl and whisk gently to combine.
3. Roughly chop the artichoke hearts into chunks.
4. Add artichokes and spinach to the egg mixture. Add all the remaining ingredients, excluding the ricotta cheese, and stir to combine.
5. Pour the mixture into the prepared dish.
6. Using a spoon, scoop the ricotta cheese onto the top of the casserole in evenly spaced dollops.
7. Place in the oven and back for 30-35 minutes, until the center of the casserole is fully cooked and does not jiggle when you shake the pan.

DAY 7

SCRAMBLED EGGS

3 tablespoons butter
1 small tomato, diced
3 large eggs
1/3 cup heavy cream
2 tablespoons cilantro, finely chopped
1/2 teaspoon salt
2 tablespoons scallions, thinly sliced
Salt and pepper, to taste

1. Place the butter in a large cast iron skillet over medium heat.
2. Add the chili and tomato and sauce for 2 minutes.
3. In a mixing bowl, whisk together the eggs, cream, cilantro, salt, and pepper.
4. Pour the egg mix into the frying pan and allow to sit for 30 seconds without touching. Then, gently lift and fold to cook the eggs. Continue until eggs are still soft, but fully cooked.
5. Sprinkle with scallions and serve warm. Enjoy!

ZUCCHINI NOODLES WITH AVOCADO CREAM SAUCE

2 large zucchini, ends trimmed and made into noodles with julienne peeler
1 avocado
1/2 cucumber, chopped
Juice of 1/2 a lemon
1 clove garlic
2 tablespoons full fat coconut milk
8 leaves of basil, roughly chopped
Salt and pepper, to taste

1. Place zucchini spirals in a large bowl.
2. In a food process, combine the remaining ingredients and process until smooth.
3. Tosh the zucchini with the avocado sauce until fully coated
4. Garnish with the basil leaves and season with salt and pepper, as desired.

Best of Luck on your Keto Way of Life: Enjoy the Ride!

It has truly been an honor to share with you these insights, inspirations, and practices that have transformed my own life, the lives of my friends and colleagues, and the lives of thousands of my patients. By adopting my keto way of life, you are transforming yourself from the inside out and the outside in. From what you eat, to how you treat yourself from the moment you wake up—remember that *gratitude attitude.* These practices will reward you with more and sustained mental and physical energy, weight-loss, reduced inflammation, greater self-esteem, more patience, more compassion, and deeper, loving, and joyful relationships with family and friends. When you bring all of these experiences together into a single moment of being you, I call this the *Mind Body Smile!* This is the gift that awaits you on your journey into the keto way of life—achieving the Mind Body Smile is my wish for you. Thank you for allowing me to be a guide along your path.

May all of your life be fertile! God Bless.

Resources

Websites:

https://mindbodysmile.com : My personal website filled with my daily inspirations and information to support you along the keto journey.

Facebook.com @CNYFertilityCenter : Here you can participate in my weekly live-streamed *Fertile Fireside Chats* where I answer questions about fertility and my keto way of life in real time.

Kendberrymd.com: Ken is a fellow myth busting western doctor, especially when it comes to a low-fat diet.

mariamindbodyhealth.com: Keto pioneer Maria Emmerich's website filled with shopping guides, helpful tips, and delicious keto recipes.

Books:

Taubes, Gary. *The Case against Sugar.* First edition. New York: Alfred A. Knopf, 2016.

Seyfried, Thomas. *Cancer as a Metabolic Disease: On the Origin, Management, and Prevention of Cancer.* First edition. Wiley, 2012

Dweck, Carol S. *Mindset: The New Psychology of Success.* New York: Ballentine, 2007

About the Author

Dr. Robert Kiltz is Founder and Director of CNY Fertility, annually ranked among the top ten fertility centers in the nation, with over 300 employees and chapters in six locations in Central New York, Atlanta and Montreal.

Over more than two decades of helping families to grow, Dr. Kiltz has developed cutting-edge approaches to fertility grounded in Western medicine and supported by practices from Eastern healing arts. To treat the whole person—mind, body, and spirit, Dr. Kiltz revolutionized the fertility industry by providing full-service Healing Arts Centers where patients receive massage, acupuncture, and yoga instruction. This patient-centered approach extends to Dr. Kiltz's commitment to democratizing access to fertility treatments by making CNY the nation's most affordable fertility clinics.

Dr. Kiltz routinely shares his thoughts on wellness, spirituality, and fertility in his blog, *Mind Body Smile,* and as host of the podcast, *The Fertile Life: Conversations with Doctor Kiltz.* Each week thousands of viewers participate in his *Fertile Fireside Chats,* broadcast live on Facebook, where he answers questions about fertility in real time, while sharing his recommendations for a ketogenic lifestyle based on a high fat, moderate protein, and low carb diet.

A thought leader in the keto movement, Dr. Kiltz believes that a keto diet dramatically improves mental clarity, fertility, and health, empowering people to live their best lives. In addition to his own media channels, Dr. Kiltz appears regularly on numerous popular blogs and has shared his views as a speaker at TEDx.

Dr. Kiltz is a Diplomat of the American Board of Obstetrics and Gynecology and Fellowship trained and Board Certified in Reproductive Endocrinology and Infertility. A Graduate of the University of Southern California, he completed medical school at the University of California, Davis. After residency at the University of Colorado Health Science Center in Denver, he practiced at Kaiser Permanente in California followed by a fellowship in Reproductive Endocrinology and Infertility at Harbor UCLA Medical Center. Prior to founding CNY Fertility, Dr. Kiltz practiced reproductive endocrinology and infertility at the Alta Bates In Vitro Fertilization Program while a clinical faculty member at the University California San Francisco, annually ranked among the top two medical schools in America.

Raised in Los Angeles, and now a Central New Yorker by choice, Dr. Kiltz is a licensed pilot, frequently commuting in his Cirrus SR22T between CNY Fertility's offices in Albany, Syracuse, Rochester, and Buffalo. He makes his home on the beautiful shores of Skaneateles Lake, where he draws inspiration from his practices as an accomplished painter and potter.

End Note

i https://www.ncbi.nlm.nih.gov/pubmed/23244540
ii https://www.eurekalert.org/pub_releases/2011-04/imc-sfr033111.php
iii https://www.ncbi.nlm.nih.gov/pmc/articles/PMC2990190/
iv https://www.ncbi.nlm.nih.gov/pubmed/23719144
v https://www.sciencedaily.com/releases/2013/10/131015123341.htm
vi https://www.ahajournals.org/doi/10.1161/CIR.0000000000000665
vii https://www.pnas.org/content/108/50/20254.full
viii https://nmr.mgh.harvard.edu/mkozhevnlab/wp-content/uploads/pdfs/Kozhevnikov_etal_meditation_2009.pdf

Made in the USA
Las Vegas, NV
19 April 2022